10-minute
Facelift

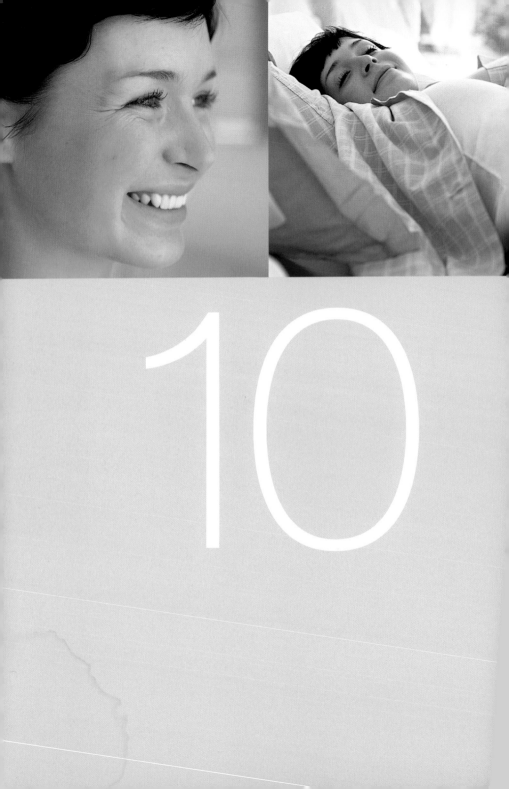

10

hamlyn

10-minute
Facelift

Tessa Thomas

For Carys

First published in Great Britain
in 2000 by Hamlyn a division of
the Octopus Publishing Group Limited,
2–4 Heron Quays, London, E14 4JP

This edition published 2004

Distributed in the United States and
Canada by Sterling Publishing Co., Inc.
387 Park Avenue South, New York,
NY 10016-8810

ISBN 0 600 61166 3

A CIP catalogue record for this book is
available from the British Library

Printed in China

Note: *Massage and facial exercise
should not be considered as a
replacement for professional medical
treatment; a physician should be
consulted in all matters relating to
health. Care should be taken during
pregnancy, particularly in the use of
essential oils and pressure points.
Essential oils should not be ingested
and should be used for babies and
children only on professional advice.*

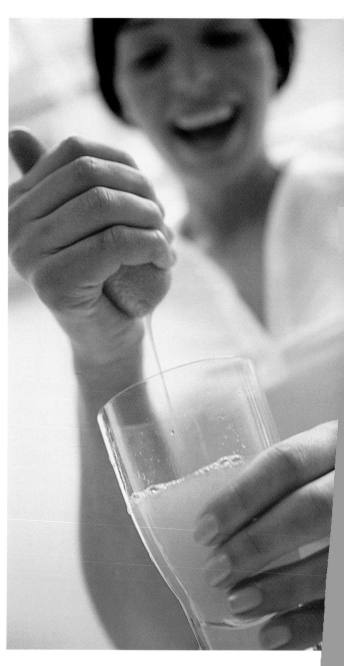

contents

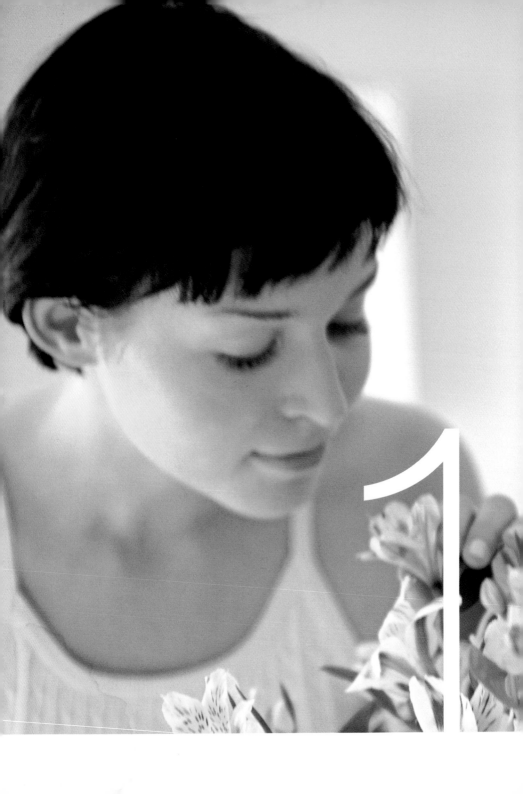

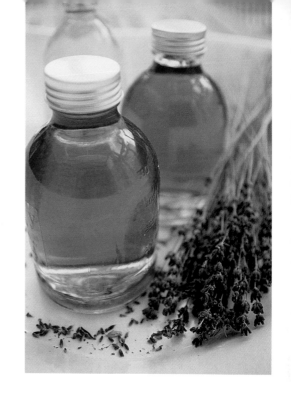

face values

face facts

Your face doesn't take up much space. Of the two square metres of skin that contours the body, that covering the face accounts for just four-and-a-half per cent. Yet it attracts more attention, generates more concern and fuels more commercial enterprise than any other part of the body. Britons spend an estimated £760 million every year on skincare products. These include sun and cellulite creams, body lotions and toners. But, despite its disproportionately small surface area, more than half of that money is spent on products for the face.

Yet the imbalance makes sense. For every face tells a story. Like the cover of a book, it announces the interior narrative. The unique features that a face develops through inheritance and experience, be they laughter lines or wilting eyes, offer myriad insights into the interior life of their wearer.

The face in culture

In some cultures its significance goes further. For the Japanese, the face contains many of the acupressure points through which energy is activated and channelled. The Chinese set store by the ancient art of 'face reading', in which the facial features and skin reflect the condition of the body's vital organs. Proponents of the Indian practice of ayurveda hold that one of the body's seven energy channels is in the jaw. Westerners may lack a formal system but they can never resist carrying out their own analysis, consciously or otherwise. 'I'm hopeless with names, but I never forget a face,' is a universal refrain.

Whatever the cultural slant, our face is interpreted as the most graphic representation of the person we have been and the one we are, in body and soul. Yet most significantly it reveals our age. As the years pass, the picture on the cover of the book is not so much sketched as etched – in wrinkles, creases, sags and bags. The most public part of our skin ages more quickly than any other.

How could it be otherwise? The skin is the body's most visible organ and the face its most exposed part. Ever open to the elements, it registers the passing of every season.

The face is also the most expressive part of the body, capable of a wider range of movements than any other, and it rarely rests. If you have found your vocation as a professional gurner or happily superannuated grandparent, the resulting wrinkles are of little concern. But if you're an ordinary mortal sensitive to the passing of time, the last thing you want is a daily reminder of its speed as you flick on the light over the bathroom mirror.

All history is written there

The furrows with which your face taunts you are now less a personal affliction, more a collective institution. As the population ages more rapidly than ever before, creases and jowls are becoming the norm. You might think that would make them more acceptable – that they may be regarded as the face of seniority, symbols of wisdom and experience. But in a world where the cult of youth reigns supreme, they signify the passing of opportunity, sexuality and beauty. The poet John Keats (1795–1821) famously asserted that beauty is truth and truth beauty: the word truth could today be substituted by youth.

So now, instead of conferring prestige, ageing skin denotes decay and senior citizens find themselves classified as wrinklies. Despite the adoption by beauty companies of older muses, even the fortysomethings are made to feel way past their aesthetic prime. No wonder American dermatologists, keen not to offend potential clients, refer to wrinkles as dermatologic corrugations.

But such euphemisms convince no one. People are flocking to clinics, chemists and beauticians in search of ready-to-wear cures. Plastic surgeons, pharmacists and laboratory technicians in cosmetics houses are the new gurus, to whom people entrust their fragile and ephemeral looks. Rejuvenation is the holy grail of the beauty industry.

Drastic measures

In the 17th century, daring women would remove their surface skin with oil of vitriol – with disastrous results. In its modern version, the facial peel – or 'resurfacing', as its polite practitioners prefer – the procedure is more scientific and controlled, but barely less painful or crude. Four centuries of preoccupation and experimentation and we have still failed, despite every effort, to discover a fail-safe facelift. But in an age of such rapid technological advance, consumers are constantly persuaded that newly synthesised chemicals, cutting-edge technology or state-of-the-art surgery will help rejuvenate their skin. Although none offers an instant or easy solution (and we know it), we are spending more than ever on all types of anti-ageing treatment, whether they involve dipping our fingers into a pot marked rejuvenating gel or undergoing days of discomfort after assault by laser.

Ultimately, neither will satisfy the self-conscious consumer, primed to expect instant results but who understands neither the skin nor the technology that promises to straighten it out. In a seductive and lucrative market that is drawing in more clients by the year, it pays to know.

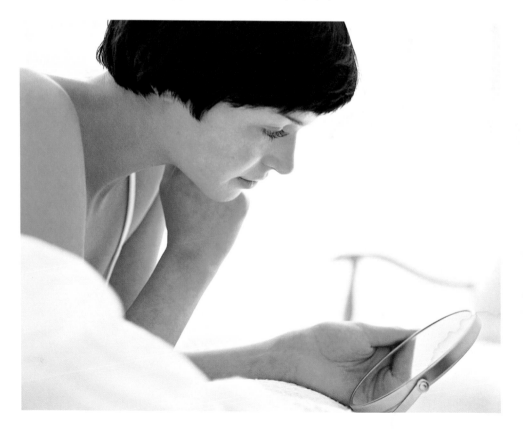

skin deep

Skin is clever stuff. It has to be. It is responsible for keeping the outside world out and the inside world in – for protecting the internal organs and retaining essential fluids while resisting infection and providing a barrier to damage.

More than a barrier

But that is not all. Your skin also regulates your body temperature by sweating when it is hot and restricting the blood supply when it is cold. It gets rid of waste materials that cannot pass through the kidneys and distributes nutrients and oxygen to the nerves, glands, hair and nails. It sends pain signals to the brain.

To do all this the skin is endowed with unique qualities. It has hair follicles to get sebum to the surface; acutely sensitive nerve receptors; elastic tissues capable of expanding by 50 per cent, and a highly productive regenerative system. It is adaptable, too, responding to one's age or mood, to the time of the month or season of the year.

As the most exposed and most expressive part of the body, your face has the body's most sophisticated skin of all. It has more nerve endings and sebaceous glands, the smallest capillaries, the thinnest skin and the finest and most flexible muscles directly attached to it.

Even within the face, these are finely specialized. The thinnest skin is found on the eyelids and lips; the thickest on the forehead, jaw and chin. The oiliest is on the nose, temples and forehead, the driest on the cheeks and jaw. No wonder people find it difficult to care for and are drawn in by the offers of help from the beauty houses.

What's in skin?

In a one-centimetre-square piece of skin there are 12 oil glands, 10 hairs, 100 sweat glands, one metre of blood vessels, 2.5 metres of nerves and a total of three million cells.

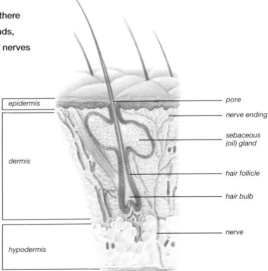

epidermis

dermis

hypodermis

pore

nerve ending

sebaceous (oil) gland

hair follicle

hair bulb

nerve

Layer upon layer

Surgeons are familiar with the inside of the skin; the rest of us know only the visible bit. But a section of skin, see diagram left, is rather like that of a herbaceous border or river-bed: the vital bits are all hidden beneath the surface.

Skin comes in multiple layers. We pamper and worry about the topmost layer, but underneath is where the real action is.

The foundation of the skin is the subcutis, a firm and spongy layer that contains fat cells, blood vessels and nerve fibres. Above that sits the dermis, which not only serves as a soft underlay for the epidermis but is also the skin's support system.

Some 3 mm thick, it contains blood vessels, nerve endings, hair follicles, oil and sweat glands and connective tissue. But most importantly perhaps, it contains collagen. Biologically, the most important role of collagen is to provide a scaffolding, holding everything together. But what it is best known for is giving the skin its bounce, vitality – and youth. Collagen production, as skincare manufacturers like to remind us, declines with age. So it is this dermal layer that is the target of every manufacturer's dream cream.

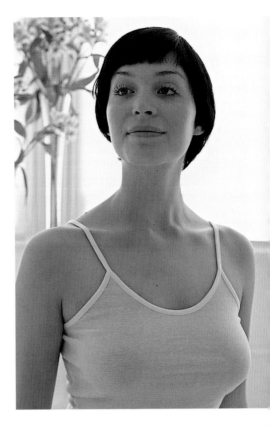

A month in the life of a skin cell

Sandwiched between the dermis and epidermis is the germinative or basal layer where the skin cells are formed. Millions are generated every day in the facial skin alone. They emerge plump and moist but immediately begin a journey to the surface during which they transform. As the cells migrate upwards, their nucleus breaks down and they fill with keratin, a tough protein that helps make them flatter and drier. All this takes around 30 days – the older you are, the longer it takes.

By the time they reach the outermost layer of the epidermis, called the stratum corneum, the cells are tough and scaly and in just the state to provide a horny, protective coating for the epidermis. After making it through the 20 layers of the stratum corneum, the cells are glued together with fatty compounds on the surface. Here they stay until they are destroyed (before their time) by detergents in cleansers or (more naturally) shed to join the dust on your household furniture.

time will tell

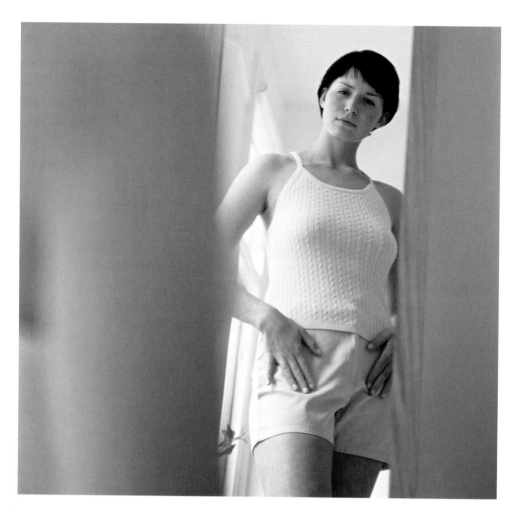

The facial skin, it is clear, has some very clever self-defence mechanisms built into it. But one thing it doesn't come with is an anti-ageing device. And as the most exposed part of the body, it is your face that ages the fastest. Every blast of cold air or ray of warm sunlight leaves its mark on your face; every puff of exhaust fumes or bottle of wine reinforces the effects that will only become more evident as time goes on.

That is all extrinsic ageing – and is partly under your control (see page 110). Then there is intrinsic ageing, which even a clean-living agoraphobe can do little about, as it is mainly determined by your genes. The combination of external and internal influences determines when you acquire an age-worn expression. In life's lucky dip, they differ from one person to another. But, all things being equal, what can you expect to happen when?

Teens

In childhood most people have skin so perfect it almost glows in the dark. Puberty marks a major transition in the skin, as it becomes oilier and more prone to blocked pores. But, pimples apart, the change is positive as the oiliness of the skin protects it from dehydration, keeping it soft and supple. Meanwhile, skin cells are regenerating with record speed, making their way from the basal layer to the epidermis in around 28 days.

Adolescence has other rewards that help compensate for the inevitable outcrop of spots. The collagen and elastin in teenage connective tissue are still perfectly cross-linked and coiled, giving it bounce and firmness. Although exposure to the sun may already have damaged the underlying tissues, that damage has not yet surfaced.

Twenties

Expression lines are beginning to form, especially between the eyebrows, at the outside corners of the eyes and across the forehead. Cell turnover is decreasing gradually and will halve over the next 25–30 years. The stratum corneum is beginning to thicken and become less flexible. The connective tissue is starting to lose its spring, especially for those who take holidays in the sun. But for all that, the facial skin still looks fresh, dewy and resilient.

Thirties

The epidermis is beginning to show visible signs of wear and tear, thanks to the cumulative effects of the sun, pollutants, stress and less-than-perfect nutrition. The resulting changes manifest themselves in an uneven complexion, dullness and retained fluid. The thickening of the stratum corneum and decrease in cell turnover are becoming more apparent. Repeated facial expressions are now pushing the fat in the subcutis into trenches which, increasingly deprived of their bounce, remain set.

Wrinkles are becoming an enduring feature and the cumulative effects of gravity are starting to show. This is when most people start to peruse the beauty counters for that anti-ageing elixir that will eradicate some of these tell-tale signs.

Forties

The journey from the basal layer to the epidermis can now take 40 days. The even patina of one's early years is disappearing as pigmentation becomes uneven, resulting for some people in dark patches. The basal layer is gradually thinning, making it more difficult for the skin cells to retain their moisture, while the stratum corneum continues to thicken. The production of sebum, which peaked in adolescence, is now in marked decline. Just as well, because there are more dead cells sticking to the skin surface as cell turnover declines. Thread veins may start to appear, especially on sensitive skin. Deepening expression lines leave no one in any doubt as to the emotional history of the wearer.

Fifties

In women, this marks the biggest change since adolescence. The menopause, which usually occurs in one's early fifties, brings a sharp decline in oestrogen production with a concomitant fall in sebum. This makes it easier for water to evaporate, leading to dry and sometimes flaky skin.

The epidermis continues to atrophy and is now about 20 per cent thinner than in one's teens. The distribution of fatty cells becomes uneven and the disproportionate number in the lower tissues leads to the emergence of drooping jowls and a heavier chin. The cumulative effects of sun exposure may manifest themselves in dark, benign patches called solar keratoses.

off-the-shelf solutions

Some people with silken skin are just luckier than others and have clearly got a choice catch from the gene pool. But even they end up looking for external help. By the age of 40, the average woman is using five creams on her face every day. The number used and the amount spent on each increases with age. They represent a form of crisis management.

Manufacturers know a growing market when they see one and with the number of older women increasing, they have responded to this crisis with a glut of anti-ageing lotions and potions. They currently account for a fifth of all facial skincare sales and the sector is growing faster than any other. But do these creams work? Many are the results of long-term research and much-publicized laboratory tests. All are ingeniously marketed. But inevitably, hope fuels hype.

Magic ingredients?

Manufacturers exploit many tactics to persuade the sceptical consumer that their latest is the cream that will, with regular use, wipe away the years even as it is applied. One of the most common tactics is the use of ingredients linked with youthful looks in the popular imagination. Vitamin E, collagen, elastin, retinol ... all are suggestively used. Even the most enlightened consumers may well confuse retinol, a form of vitamin A, with retinoic acid. But while the latter – a powerful prescription drug – does eliminate wrinkles, retinol will do no such thing. Similarly, although collagen injections can plump out creases and young skin is rich in elastin, collagen and elastin in a cream simply cannot be absorbed into the dermis. Ditto vitamin E – an additive with a sting in its tail, as it can also cause contact dermatitis.

Hidden dangers

Not all new ingredients call the consumer's bluff. Liposomes, for example, do just what the manufacturers say: they transport moisture into the skin and trap it there. But at what chemical cost? If synthetic ingredients such as these are absorbed on contact with the skin – and by some estimates more than 50 per cent are – then there is every chance some enter the bloodstream and get transported to the liver. Beauty companies may test their preparations for allergic reactions on the skin but the true effects may be much deeper down.

Although the permitted amount of each ingredient is small, there is no limit to the number of chemicals that can be incorporated into a single product. By one estimate, two kilos of cosmetic chemicals find their way into the average user's bloodstream every year. Furthermore, while the effects of individual constituents have been tested, little account is taken of the 'cocktail effect' that may result when these chemicals are combined.

But the effects are hidden and their origin impossible to prove. Not so when people get adverse reactions to a facial product on their skin. Complaints about such reactions have increased with the range, aims and claims of products. Hardly surprising that 80 per cent of women questioned in one survey said they have sensitive skin.

In a recent trial of anti-ageing creams by the Consumers' Association, more than a third of the 48 women reported effects on their skin such as burning, itching, flakiness and dryness. Yet such is the belief that treatment for skin is a patented, processed and packaged product, the usual response is to buy another cream to put right the after-effects of the last – and so the cycle continues.

Beauty by nature?

The rise in sales of organic food and low-chemical household cleaners is paralleled by an increase in so-called 'natural' skincare products. One of the marketing buzzwords of recent years, 'natural' is also one of the most abused – and nowhere more so than on the beauty counters.

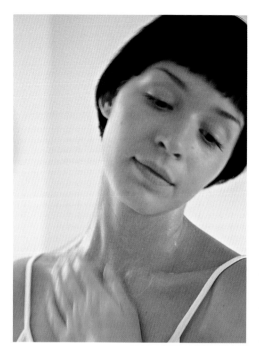

Water. You couldn't get more natural than that. But water provides the perfect medium for fungal and bacterial growth, so necessitates the addition of preservatives – which are invariably synthetic. The use of chemicals requires the inclusion of perfumes to disguise their smells. Yet perfumes, which are made up from a potential range of more than 600 chemicals, are responsible for more adverse skin reactions than any other component in face creams.

Of course, the secondary effects of artificial chemicals can be reduced by decreasing the amount in the product. This has happened with fruit acids, which have come a long way since the Romans plastered the residue of fermented grape skins over their faces. The modern processed versions used in clinics are infinitely stronger (see table on page 19). But even the diluted over-the-counter versions were the target of so many complaints when they were launched that their makers were forced to reduce the amount of fruit acid in creams to a barely effective 2–5 per cent.

Beauty at what price?

While the effect of these creams and other 'anti-ageing' preparations are at best minimal and at worst questionable, the cost can be astronomical. A single pot can set you back more than £50; some carry a price tag in the hundreds. Breathtaking promises command mind-boggling prices.

They are worth paying if the feeling of being pampered takes years off you, but do it knowing two things. First, that the 'active ingredients' constitute only around five per cent of the product (with much of the remaining cost going into the pretty packaging and alluring advertising). Second, that the effect of any cosmetic preparation is by definition temporary. Only a drug, which comes under different regulations and has to be licensed, can legitimately claim to effect an enduring change on your skin or any other organ.

A manufacturer can legitimately claim their product is scented with a 'natural' fragrance even if the essential oil it contains accounts for just one per cent of the product and synthetic scents are also used. They can highlight the inclusion in a cream of natural wheatgerm, avocado or evening primrose oil when these are made from genetically modified plants – the unknown effects of which have caused the more ethical (and genuinely natural) skincare manufacturers to ban GMO ingredients. They can refer to elastin as a natural ingredient, even when it is derived from animal tissue and so highly chemically preserved. They can emphasize the inclusion of vitamin C because it is necessary for collagen production, even though collagen in the dermis is untouched by vitamin C in a cream.

And despite all these magical ingredients, what is the most common constituent of skin creams?

chemistry versus surgery

Since 1997, beauty companies have been legally obliged to list the contents of their products. But you may need degrees in Latin and pharmacology to understand them, as they use a rarefied Latinate 'Eurolanguage'. This not only blurs the distinction between natural and synthetic ingredients but carries no reference to the origin or effect of the chemicals contained.

Beware of long lists and names. One leading dermatologist warns that if a product says it contains more than three active ingredients, it cannot live up to its claims; another that if you can't pronounce the names of the ingredients, suspect that they may do you as much harm as good.

More than 3,000 chemicals are licensed for use in cosmetic products in Europe. Many are anodyne, some are not. Watch out for the following:

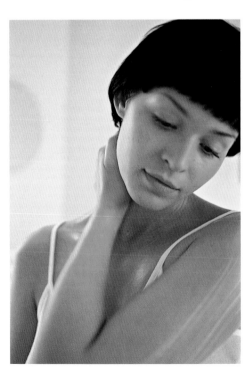

Propylene glycol: a clear liquid designed to carry moisture, it is a very common skin allergen.

Sodium lauryl sulphate: a detergent, emulsifier and wetting agent, it often dries the skin and is a common form of irritant because it eats into the skin protein.

Diethanolamine (DEA) and triethanolamine (TEA): wetting agents that can form nitrosamines, which are potentially carcinogenic, and formaldehyde, which not only is highly allergenic but can cause gene mutations in animals and has been banned in Japan and Sweden. Other chemicals, such as the preservatives 2-bromo-2-nitropropane-1, 3-diol (commonly called bronopol), can have a similar effect.

Parabens or parabenz: a preservative used in a third of cosmetics, its suspected carcinogenic potential has led to its being banned in Japan. Parabens are found in nature but most cosmetics manufacturers use the synthesized forms, known as butyl, ethyl, methyl or propyl parabens.

Parahydroxy benzoates: preservatives and anti-fungal agents which cause allergic reactions and on which a ban has been proposed in the US.

Imidazolidinyl urea (also called hydantoin): used to synthesize lubricants, it is derived from wood alcohol, which can cause nausea, and is carcinogenic in animals. Can also produce formaldehyde.

Stearic acid: a waxy fatty acid often used in skin creams, it frequently causes sensitivity.

Lanolin: derived from sheep's wool, it may contain carcinogenic pesticides which could be carried into the bloodstream as lanolin is fat-soluble.

Quaternium 15: a common cause of contact dermatitis in chemically sensitive people.

Boric acid: a bactericide and fungicide used in skin fresheners, it can cause toxic reactions. Talcum powder containing boric acid carries a warning that it is not to be used on the under-3s.

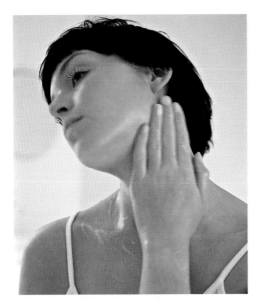

Whatever the reason, people are more prepared than ever to undergo days or weeks of discomfort and isolation to burn, peel or sand the years off their face. Youth comes at a cost in more ways than one, but people are increasingly prepared to pay it.

The demand has been fuelled by new techniques, from laser treatment to dermabrasion. However, most do not stand the test of time and need to be repeated within a year or two. And so to the operating theatre.

Record numbers of people – mainly, but not all, women – are entrusting their looks to cosmetic surgeons. By one estimate, 65,000 people (in the UK) go under the knife each year, though the real figure is certainly higher since many such operations are carried out in unlicensed clinics. Far more people think of doing so. One study in 1999 suggested that one in four women under 40 were considering cosmetic surgery. Doubtless many will be put off before they reach the operating table by the consultant's description of the gory procedure in store (see table on page 19).

If you are of sturdier spirit than these and still considering such treatment, turn first to page 46. Doing facial exercises before a cosmetic operation can significantly improve and prolong the result.

Benzyl alcohol: a common preservative in creams, it is a frequent cause of hypersensitivity.
Butylated hydroxy anisole (Bha) and Butylated hydroxy toluene (Bht): commonly used antioxidants that can cause delayed hyper-sensitivity with regular use.
Tocopherol and tocopherol acetate: commonly used antioxidants that can cause contact dermatitis.
Blue 1 and green 3: artificial colours, they are both carcinogenic.

A last resort

The blitz of new creams hitting the cosmetics counters in recent times has not stemmed the tide of people seeking radical solutions. Perhaps the creams don't work as promised; perhaps people want a quick fix; perhaps they can't resist the temptation of a new technique; or perhaps they are just after a deeper and more lasting effect – some long-term intensive care rather than peremptory, and temporary, first-aid.

what's the alternative?

Operations and preparations that claim to iron out wrinkles, lift up bags or plump out creases are sorely tempting. They appeal to our vanity and indolence. But they are, like make-up, a short-term cover-up. If you have an old wooden table whose original allure has faded with use, you can sand and varnish, then dust and polish it regularly. But if you overlook the hairline crack in a leg, the table will eventually deteriorate beyond repair.

If the crack is noticed soon enough, you can take action – to fill it in, cover it with veneer or remodel the leg. Similarly, you can have your wrinkles filled out with collagen, covered with new skin after a peel or ironed out with a partial or full facelift. The pros and cons of the most common cosmetic procedures are shown in the table opposite.

Pre-emptive action

But how much better to care for the underlying structure in the first place, prevent cracks or creases appearing and preserve the natural foundation. For the face, that means two key things: keeping the muscles fit and strong, and allowing the connective tissue around them to relax and remain supple.

A huge range of machines is marketed claiming to do both for you. They come in all forms, from vibrating goggles for home use to low-frequency electric probes manipulated by a beautician. But

equally good – and more enduring – effects are achieved with some self-tuition and daily care at home. All you need is a pair of hands, a spot of oil, a mirror and some dedication.

If facial massage and exercise are all you do, you will keep your looks longer than most. But add to them an internal spring-clean and a diet that feeds your skin, and your complexion will bloom. Water it regularly outside and in to keep it that way.

A ten minute workout

It will take no more than ten minutes a day and could take as many years off you. You can also save the hours once spent perusing beauty counters for that elusive anti-wrinkle cream or firming gel that promised to cover up the tracks of time.

Instead of buying a foundation cream to conceal your skin, build a natural foundation with well-toned muscle. Instead of putting energy into looking for the ultimate crow's feet cream, put it into eye exercises. Instead of buying a new blusher brush, achieve a rosy glow by boosting your circulation. Instead of paying for a high-tech moisturizer, turn on the kitchen tap. And rather than covering creases, smooth them away with some gentle massage.

There will always be other things you could usefully do in that time; mow a lawn, dust the furniture, make a meal. But none of their effects will endure. Spend the time on five minutes of exercise, four of massage and a one-minute cleanse and the results will still be looking back at you from the mirror next year.

If you follow this programme, you won't have the luxury of feeling pampered and you won't have any glitzy packaging to brighten your bathroom shelf. But you might have an enviable complexion that belies your age. 'All beauty fades and ugliness endures – except that of the skin,' the poet and author Edith Sitwell wrote. Here's your chance to prove her wrong.

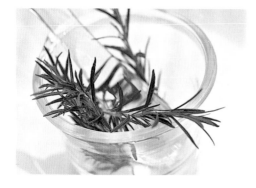

What happens	Advantages	Disadvantages
A **Facelift** is when the skin is cut and lifted, then draped back over the face and the excess cut off. The muscles can be lifted and lightened at the same time. Parts of certain muscles can also be lifted to prevent further furrowing and creasing of the face.	Improves the shape of the face and removes surface lines. Once the bruising and scarring have faded, the improvement is immediately visible and will last six to ten years. Where certain areas of the face are particularly affected, a smaller operation can be performed – most typically a browlift or eyelift.	If the procedure is repeated, facial mobility is reduced so the face is less expressive. Carries a small risk of nerve damage, which may be permanent. Results in a mask-like effect if the skin is stretched taut when lifted. The surface area of the skin is reduced so it may be less efficient at circulating essential nutrients and air.
Laser Treatment is used to remove the eperdimis and part of the dermis with a high-powered beam of energy.	Can be very closely targeted for individual wrinkles and the depth of the ablation accurately controlled with the use of magnifying instruments. Works well fine wrinkles such as crow's feet and upper lip wrinkles.	Skin is painful, swollen and covered in a crust for up to ten days and pink for 3–6 months before it resumes its natural colour. Risk of irregular pigmentation, especially if skin is regularly exposed to sun. Not very effective on deep furrows. Sensitivity to cosmetics may be increased. Demarcation line may be visible if not expertly done.
Dermabrasion is when a rotating wire brust or diamond wheel removes the epidermis and top part of the dermis, removing fine lines and wrinkles. The abraded skin regrows thicker, with new collagen and elastin.	Effective on deep upper-lip wrinkles.	Same disadvantages as laser treatment, with added disadvantage that dermabrasion produces more bleeding and the new look of the skin lasts only a matter of months.
Chemical peeling is the application of an abrasive acid paste to the face, which removes the epidermis. New skin regrows as above.	Can be done with different pastes and to varying depths according to severity of wrinkles. Lightest and most popular is the alpha-hydroxy (fruit) acid peel, which is very quick and less painful but the results of which are less dramatic. A phenol peel is more effective but often reduces pigmentation.	Paste has to be applied about three times over 24 hours. Removal of paste is very painful. Skin is red, flaky and swollen for up to a month after a light peel, several months after a deep one. Destroys surface pigment cells, so exposure to sun can cause pigmentation problems. Not good for neck, which heals poorly.
Collagen implantation is the injection of animal collagen into wrinkles. The lines are filled out immediately and the body's own production of natural collagen stimulated over the subsequent months.	There is no scarring and the improvement is immediate, though red spots may be visible for a few hours after treatment.	Lasts a few months at most. Often requires course of up to three injections. Possibility of allergic reaction. Need to avoid using facial muscles for around four hours after treatment.
Fat implantation is the removal of fat from the stomach or thigh under local anasthetic. Blood and excess fluid is removed and fat cells injected. Collagen grows around the new fat.	Good for deep wrinkles. No risk of allergic reaction.	A lot of fat cells need to be implanted, making the face red and lumpy for several weeks or even some months. More expensive than silicone or collagen, though a lot of the fat will disappear.
Silicone injection is the injection of silicone deep into wrinkles. The body produces collagen that surrounds the silicone, filling out the wrinkle.	Effect is permanent as silicone remains in tissue. Good for forehead and mouth furrows.	Risk of silicone migrating to other parts of the body, so many practitioners no longer offer the treatment, which has been outlawed in the US.
Botox 'hibernation' is the injection of botulism toxin into the muscle to paralyse it, so creases cannot deepen.	Very effective for forehead lines. Most often used on frowning muscles.	Limits expression in face. Only lasts 3–4 months.

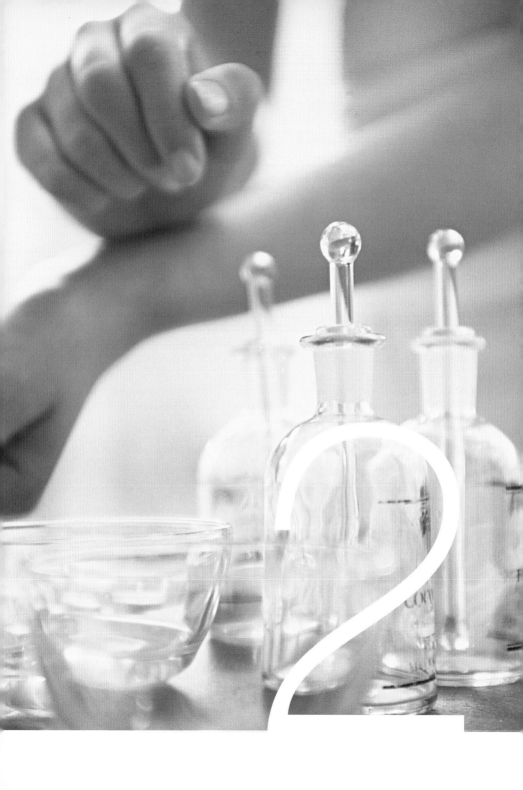

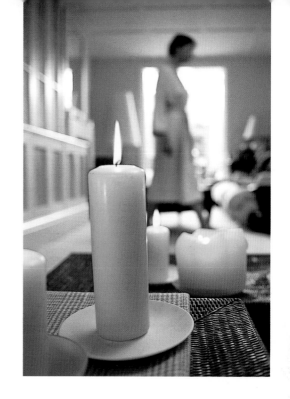

getting in touch

meridians and magic

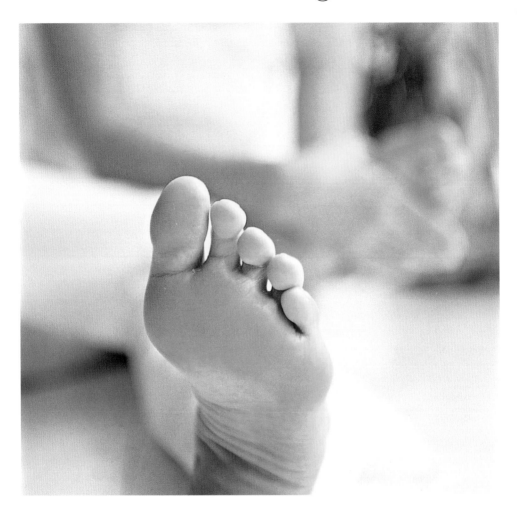

Trap your finger in the door and the first thing you do, after swearing, is to hold it firmly. Pick up a child who has tripped over and your instinct is to rub the knee or elbow she has bashed. If a cat decides to nestle into your lap, all but the acutely allergic will instinctively stroke it.

Touch is a primitive instinct and one that derives from the concrete physical benefits it confers. When you press or squeeze a part of your body, it increases circulation to that area. When one person holds another with sensitivity, they relax.

Yet we rarely touch our faces at all. You may find yourself half-consciously picking a spot or, in a moment of alarm, pressing a hand against your forehead. But rarely do we touch our own face in a nurturing way. Rather, we treat it as an ornamental object on which we carry out various decorative or preservative rituals. So we know it intimately by sight – often all too intimately. But if technology were able to present people with an exact replica of their face to identify by touch, few would be able to identify it as their own.

This is a pity because, like other parts of the body, the face responds well to touch. Better, in fact, because it is so packed with small, sensitive muscles and so richly endowed with nerve endings. If you feel a tap on the shin, you may not be sure whether it was the errant toecap of the person seated opposite or the leg of the table. But any contact with your face immediately registers its strength and form. So if it is touched sensitively, your face will respond positively.

Healing hands

Like the face, the fingertips are also exceptionally well supplied with nerve endings that give them an acute sensitivity. Many masseurs believe that the hands are specially endowed to transmit the body's magnetic force – something that the traditional medicines of the east regard as a healing force. So the hands and face go together make a perfect therapeutic team.

According to the principles of traditional Chinese medicine, it goes further than that – to your toes if you like. Under the system of acupressure the body is seen to have a network of energy channels called meridians. At strategic points along the meridians are points that are the keys to releasing energy. Running up and down the body, many meridians end in the feet and many in the face; both key points of sensual contact.

So there are a number of ways in which touch can act as a release for the face. But if ageing skin is your main concern then it is the effect which touch can have on the connective tissue which you will be most interested in.

The connective tissue sits between the layers of the dermis and the muscle (see diagram on page 10). Richer in elastic fibres than connective tissue in other parts of the body, it should be flexible and stretchy. But tension, and to a certain extent age, cause it to become less supple. The spaces between the connective fibres are filled with a gelatin-like 'ground substance'. As time goes on, the chains of molecules that form this substance get bound together and as these are less flexible than shorter links, the gelatin substance becomes both harder and stiffer.

This has a knock-on effect on the muscles, which have less room to move. A decrease in muscle mobility has four negative effects:
• First, it means the muscles are less able to extend and relax.
• Second, it constricts their possibilities for exercise. This is why, if tension is a problem (and who escapes it these days?), facial massage should precede facial exercise.
• Third, muscular rigidity encourages habitual expressions to set in as part of the fabric of the face. Life in the 21st century is such that those expressions are often of stress and strain – the very ones that pull the tissues downward and age the sppearance of our faces.
• Fourth, rigidity in the connective tissue most affects the finest muscles, such as those that control the movement of the eyes and lips. These are just the areas that are covered with the thinnest skin and have fewest sebaceous glands, so wrinkle most rapidly whatever face you pull or suppress.

By loosening up the connective tissue, light facial massage can create more space for the muscles to exercise and to relax (see fingertip facelift on page 120).

changing faces

People hold the tension in different parts of their faces, the most common being the jaw, forehead and eyes. Sometimes it is so marked that it is immediately visible: a permanently retracted or jutting chin, a raised or furrowed brow and squinting or half-closed eyes are the most typical examples. So it is small surprise that among the most common complaints in later years are jowls and double chins, frown lines and creased brows, and droopy lids and crow's feet.

Storing tension

But tension can be stored in or around anyone's facial features: it depends on your personality, life-long habits and even your profession. It is when this tension is repeatedly locked in the same place for years that it etches into the skin the lines that reflect your attitudes, your history – and your age. The earlier you become aware of where you bury your anxieties, the easier it will be to minimize the effects on your skin (see right).

Tension and stress are difficult to avoid: the person who rarely knits their brows is either exceptionally lucky or chemically tranquilized. But as gentle pressure loosens up the muscles and gives them room for manoeuvre, they learn to slide back into place more readily after being tensed. The creases and furrows then have less opportunity to engrave themselves in the skin.

As soon as you expunge some of the residual tension from the face, your complexion brightens and your expression lightens. And, as with any physical or psychological therapy, the effect is cumulative, such that with repeated self-treatments the years will roll back a little.

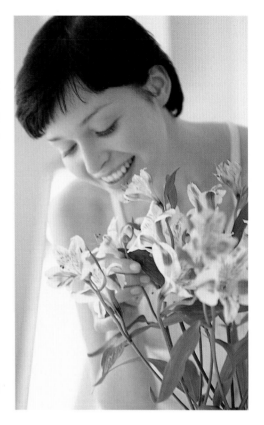

Being aware of tension in the face

Although you cannot erase the causes of tension in everyday life, you can increase your awareness of them. Most of us knit our brows, grit our teeth or purse our lips unconsciously. One reason these expressions leave their mark so dramatically on the skin is that we do them many times in the average day without realizing.

By becoming more aware of what your face is doing, you can reduce the time these muscles are tensed and limit the damage to the skin.

There will also be a psychological pay-off. As practitioners of many complementary therapies would confirm, there is an intimate reciprocal relationship between the way we use our bodies and the emotions we feel. Replace frowns with smiles and, even if this is done with some effort of will, it will affect the release of mood-enhancing brain chemicals such as endorphins and serotonin. If you have a ton of work to do and a deadline that looks impossible, smiling isn't easy, but even releasing your frown can help.

As with any behaviour that goes against what you would naturally do, it helps to have a few techniques you can call on. Try any of the following:

• When you feel your face tense up, ask yourself what purpose your anxiety or anger is serving. If your feelings are merited, act on them and get rid of them. If not, breathe deeply and concentrate on your breathing. Try to turn your mind to the next positive thing on your agenda.

• Watch other people and note their unconscious facial contortions. Whether they are standing in a shop queue, hurrying for the bus or carrying a heavy case, most will be negative ones. Observing their expressions should help you become more aware of your own.

• If all else fails, stick a piece of tape over the skin between your eyebrows. You won't be able to frown without its crinkling, creasing or peeling, bringing the fact to your attention.

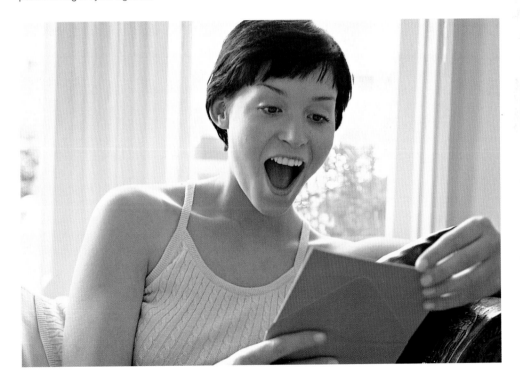

on the move

Look in the mirror when you first get up in the morning, if you dare. What do you see? A face that probably looks paler, puffier and more creased than usual. Some of the creases you can blame on the pillow you have slept on; but the lack of colour and tone have little to do with your bed linen. They are the result of a nocturnal slow-down in circulation.

When the body is in deep rest it slows the systems that pump blood and lymph around the body. The heartbeat slows, blood pressure falls and lymph flow drops to a comparative trickle.

Lymph

Although it is given far less attention than blood circulation, that of the lymph is critical to health and a major influence on the condition of the skin. While the blood vessels transport nutrients and oxygen around the body, the lymph vessels carry away the waste. They work as a sort of an internal drainage system, removing toxins from the tissues.

At night, when the drainage slows down, the waste builds up. Puffiness in the face, particularly around the eyes, in the morning is just one of the most obvious signs; likewise, the relative pallor that follows the nocturnal slow down in blood circulation.

But it is not only sleep that slows circulation down. During the day, lack of exercise, poor nutrition, shallow breathing and overexposure to pollution – all hazards of modern living – slow the drainage of lymph and flow of blood.

Massage jump-starts both. A pinker glow is the testament to improved blood flow. An acceleration in lymph action is less visible, but if your face is a richer colour the lymph has also been stimulated, since its vessels run closer to the surface of the skin (see page 76-7). In the longer term, a fluid lymph system shows in a resilient immune system and a bright complexion. Half of the lymph nodes in the body are in the neck, so unblocking them has an immediate effect on the facial skin.

A gentle touch

The muscles of the face are extremely delicate. This is because, with the exception of the frontalis muscle across the forehead (see page 53), they are tethered to the bone only at one end; the other end is attached to the connective tissue and muscle. The muscle under the eye that contracts when you squint, for example, is attached to bone at the top but then runs into skin tissue at the bottom.

By contrast, elsewhere in the body, muscles are attached at both ends, giving them a firmer base that makes them more resilient. Muscles in the calf or forearm can brace tightly, whereas those in the face cannot. It is this very flexibility and freedom that give the facial muscles such an extraordinary range of expression. But it also means that, if pulled too hard or too often, the facial muscles are more susceptible to being overstretched. Massage can be tremendously beneficial to them. But if given too deeply or frequently, it can encourage the muscles to lengthen.

Losing your elasticity

That isn't a problem for young muscles: as strong and flexible as new rubber bands, they snap back into their original form with vigorous force when stretched. But elasticity of the skin, though it varies from one person to another, is always eroded by time. At varying rates, the facial muscle inevitably becomes more like the dried-up, brittle elastic band found in the bottom of an office drawer.

When stretched to its limits, that band will not only fail to regain its original taut form but possibly snap. Similarly, with age the stretchy fibres in the connective tissue and muscle become less resilient. Although they are designed to expand, if they are overstretched they can eventually tear. Although this is not painful, it is irreparable. Other fibres that interlace with the ruptured one will continue to do their job, so there is little actual loss of movement.

But tone is visibly lost. These tiny ruptures in the underlying tissue show up as lines on the surface.

So the comparative fragility of older muscles and their adjacent tissues is important to bear in mind when handling the facial skin of adults. The scalp is a different matter and can be massaged quite vigorously without any harm, with many benefits for the face (see page 123).

Sensitive skin, which is typically fair and dry, should also be massaged with great care. It is more susceptible to the kind of surface damage that causes 'broken veins' (which are not actually broken, but simply closer than usual to the surface, so more visible). Also, if heavy oil is used for massaging sensitive skin it can penetrate the fine pores deeply, clogging them and leaving them open.

Additional benefits of massage

A light touch when massaging has another benefit. It stimulates the parasympathetic nervous system. This is the system that triggers functions associated with relaxation: slow breathing, lowered blood pressure, a measured heart-beat, decreased circulation of adrenalin and the production of mood-enhancing endorphins.

So, apart from any direct effect on tensed-up facial tissues, delicate massage can have immediate psychological benefits that extend throughout the body. It is not unusual for the recipient to drift off and even fall asleep.

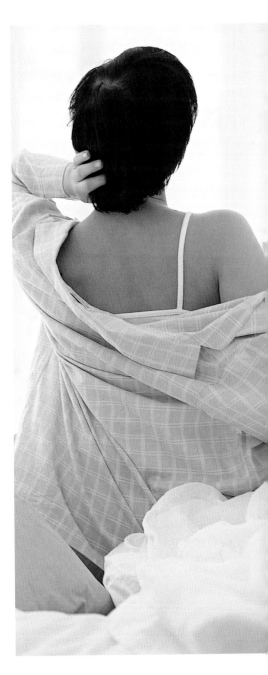

the massage environment

Massage should work on tension in body and soul, offering a simultaneous release on both levels. You can maximize the effects of a massage by creating an environment that is conducive to emotional and physical relaxation.

This does not necessarily mean draping the windows in kaftan curtains, drenching the air with heavy incense and playing native Indian music. Although these clichéd mood-makers can work for some people, there is nothing special about them. They are simply methods of appealing to the parasympathetic nervous system, so that your mind and body slow down.

What is important is that you discover the environment in which you massage more sedating than stimulating. There are four main influences:

Lighting One reason that people find it easier to sleep at night than in the day is that gloom, as its figurative meaning suggests, is a mild depressant. It acts on the hypothalamus, a primitive part of the brain, to decrease alertness. The eyeball is also a key point of tension in the face. If it is not relaxed – which it rarely is, as it picks up and sends messages

to the brain more quickly than any other sense organ – then other associated muscles are stressed. So if you are doing your massage in the day, draw the curtains. If at night, have no more than a single side-light on.

Sound Noise is a powerful nervous stimulant and raises the levels of adrenalin in the blood. In fact, studies have shown a parallel increase in the power and frequency of environmental noise and stress-related ailments over the past 15 years. So ideally you should do your massage in the quietest room in the house. But that does not preclude music, which can be a powerful tranquillizer.

Smell Odour works directly on the limbic system; this is a primitive part of the brain that operates unconsciously. To have no dominant smell is better than to have a foul one. But create one that has a tranquillizing effect and you can enhance the relaxing effects of a massage.

The most effective way to create a relaxing environment is to burn essential oil in the room. A wide range of oils that have tranquilizing effects and cater to all tastes is available. Smell is a very individual thing and some you may find utterly distasteful. Those most popular among masseurs include lavender, bergamot, petitgrain, sandalwood and ylang ylang (see pages 34–5). You can also choose from a range of burners, from a simple metal ring that rests on a light bulb to ornate stones.

Temperature Centrally heated houses are often too warm. They not only encourage sluggish blood circulation but also dry out the skin. Generally, homes should not be heated above 65°C. The main exception is when you massage. If you are not warm, your muscles will find it difficult to relax. If you do not have central heating, wear warm clothes, though not bulky ones on top. Although it is not

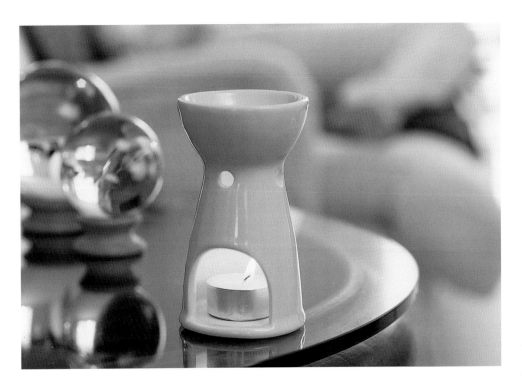

sexy, thermal underwear is a most efficient form of portable personal heating.

Despite all its proven benefits, massage alone – whether eastern or western, vigorous or delicate – will not rejuvenate your face. Like every other part of the body, to retain its youthful vigour, the face has to be exercised.

Making massage work

• Before you start, wash and warm your hands (rubbing them together heats them quickly).
• Get everything prepared before you start: mix your oil if using a blend or adding essential oils. Take off enough clothes to enable you to massage your neck and shoulders easily, and preferably wrap a towel around your body.

• If you are using oil, always pour it on to your hands first, not directly on to your face.
• Always massage with an upward and outward circular motion, so as not to drag the muscles down.
• Apply a gentle pressure so that your fingers move over the skin. If you feel your skin moving over the muscle or bone, you are pressing too hard.
• Use a small amount of oil or your fingers will slip about and lose the sensitive contact they need with the skin.

go on,oil yourself!

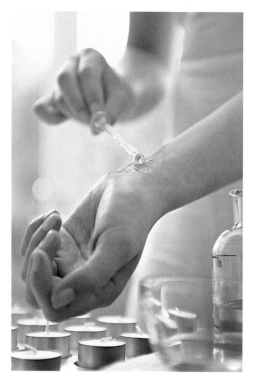

Plant oils have always been one of the essentials in the beauty box. The ancient Egyptians smeared their faces with everything from castor-berry to lettuce oil, kept in elaborate coloured glass vials. The Elizabethans imported buffalo oil, while the more conservative Victorians made copious use of almond oil, an age-old favourite that is still widely used – though fortunately the less well-off among us are no longer advised to use mutton suet as a cheap substitute.

What all these oils have in common is that they are as likely to be used in the kitchen as in the bathroom. Pure vegetable oils can nourish and lubricate the skin in a way that others cannot, as they are more efficiently absorbed and warm the skin to maximize absorption.

They cannot replace the skin's natural oils, which inexorably diminish with age: you need to ensure you have enough oils in your diet to keep those topped up (see page 95). But natural plant oils can condition the skin and, to an extent, slow down its dehydration by reducing the escape of moisture. Although any oil can block the pores of skin that is very fine or over-handled, vegetable oils do not spread a suffocating film over the skin or adversely affect its own oil production.

Oil and massage

Oil is thought to be an integral ingredient for massage. The one part of the body for which it is not always true is the face. Some people produce enough oil from their sebaceous glands to allow the fingers to slide smoothly on what is a very small surface area. Others have sensitive skin and oiling can overheat the delicate tissues, causing the pores to open too wide. Some masseurs also argue that using oil decreases the sensitive contact between fingers and face.

If used in massage, the main purpose of an oil is simply to provide a fine, slippery surface so that the skin is not pulled and stretched as you handle it. In principle, any vegetable or nut oil will do this. But if you want to make the most of their different cosmetic properties at the same time, choose from the lists on page 35 those which will best nourish and condition your skin type.

All natural oils can remove the day's grime from the skin without abrasion, simultaneously lubricating it. So using these oils for a facial massage can become part of your everyday cleansing or moisturizing routine.

Vegetable or mineral?

Commercial oils tend to have a largely mineral or vegetable composition. Although both are 'natural' in that they are the product of naturally occurring materials, they have very different qualities and effects on the skin.

Mineral oils These are not absorbed by the skin. Instead, they sit like a thin plastic film on the surface of the epidermis. This blocks the pores by 40–60 per cent, depriving the skin of vital oxygen. While it may slow down the evaporation of water from the skin, it will also stop sweat escaping as readily as it should. In the short term, the result is blackheads and blemishes. In the longer term, the skin's ability to produce its own oils will be reduced.

Mineral oils do not, like vegetable and nut oils, contain any nutrients to benefit the skin. However, they are popular with skincare manufacturers because they rarely produce allergic reactions, are cheap to produce and have a long shelf-life.

As living products, vegetable and nut oils by contrast do go rancid, especially if left open to the air. But their oxidation can be postponed, if not prevented, by adding to them vitamin E oil, which is a natural antioxidant.

Vegetable oils These have other benefits. As well as protecting the skin without blocking the pores, they contain fatty acids and fat-soluble vitamins. Many are absorbed relatively slowly by the skin, so take effect over time. However, many commercial vegetable oils are hot-pressed, a process that destroys their nutrients; so go for cold-pressed, which are usually sold in health shops.

Some vegetable oils are better suited to certain skin types than others. Broadly speaking, the drier your skin the more it will benefit from an oil rich in saturated fatty acids. Being thicker and stickier, these are absorbed more slowly and curb water loss more effectively. Greasier skins require oils with a high percentage of polyunsaturated fats, which are thinner and quickly absorbed into the skin.

If you are not sure of your skin type (dry, normal or oily), give your skin a break for a week. Go without moisturizers or make-up and cleanse only with water and the mildest cleansing bar and the true nature of your skin will be revealed. It may be that your toner is drying out your skin, your moisturizer clogging your pores or your foundation producing irritation.

Once you have decided on your skin type try one of the carrier oils from pages 32–3 which suits you and choose an essential oil from the table on page 35 to perfume it.

Warning *Always use essential oils with care. There are few oils that can be used in their undiluted form so always dilute them unless there is a specific instruction to use them in their neat form.*

Before using an oil, always check that it is safe for you. If you have a pre-existing medical condition, are receiving medical treatment, taking homoeopathic treatment, are pregnant or breastfeeding, or have sensitive skin or a skin condition, do not use the oils until you have checked with your medical adviser and a fully trained aromatherapist.

Always carry out a patch test first to check that your skin will not react adversely to the oil. Place a diluted drop on the skin. Leave on for 24 hours. If you see any adverse reaction such as reddening, scaling or any other disturbance of skin texture, DO NOT USE.

skin types

When giving yourself a facial massage, choose an oil to suit your skin type.

Dry or ageing skin

Apricot oil, which is extracted from the kernel of the fruit, is easily absorbed into the skin and has a softening effect. It has a mild fragrance and a calming effect on irritated skin.

Avocado oil is made from the dried flesh of the fruit, so is rich in nutrients, including vitamins D, E and B5, and helps restore damaged skin tissue.

Macadamia oil, made from the nuts, is made up of 40 per cent saturated acids, but is quite easily absorbed by the skin. It has a soft and silky feel and traps in a lot of moisture.

Wheatgerm oil is a very dark yellow, sticky oil with a prominent smell that needs to be blended with a less potent oil. It is often recommended for ageing skin because it is rich in minerals and vitamin E. Despite this, it does oxidize quickly and may need more vitamin E added to stop it going rancid.

Normal skin

Olive oil is one of the thicker vegetable oils, so can be mixed with thinner oils for use in massage. It contains polyunsaturated fatty acids that can help treat inflamed or scarred skin. But its pungent smell is not to everyone's taste.

Almond oil is an old favourite, used since antiquity in skincare. It is light, pleasantly scented, spreads

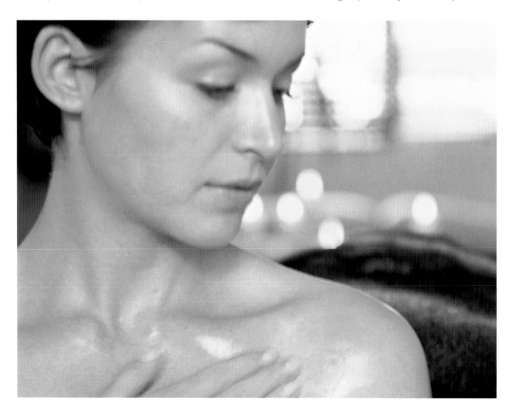

well and is easily absorbed, so is good for massage. It also mixes well with borage or macadamia for dry or ageing skin.

Sunflower oil is made from the flower's seeds and contains a lot of linoleic acid, which helps to keep the skin supple. It spreads and is absorbed easily, so can be mixed with fattier oils, such as jojoba or wheatgerm, to stop them creating a greasy film on the skin surface.

Sesame oil is a semi-fat oil that can be used for most skin types. More often found in the wok than on the cosmetics shelf, it has nevertheless long been used as a sun oil and hair oil. It is mild and can even be used around the eyes, but its pungent aroma means it is usually diluted with a more moderate oil, such as sunflower or safflower.

Oily skin

Hazelnut oil is easily absorbed and slightly astringent. It regulates sebum production, so can help normalize oily skin.

Peach kernel oil is similar to apricot but less sticky and so suits more oily skins. It contains vitamins A and E and penetrates the skin well.

Thistle oil is thin and runny, so is easily absorbed and does not block the pores. It contains up to 80 per cent linoleic acid, which helps to keep skin supple and well hydrated.

Hypericum oil is made by macerating hypericum flowers in olive oil. The flowers release hypericum, which is used medicinally as an antidepressant and gives the oil a mildly astringent quality. Hypericum needs to be blended with another carrier oil.

Two oils that deserve a special mention for their anti-ageing properties are **borage** and **evening primrose.** They are both rich in gamma-linoleic acid (GLA), which has been found to strengthen skin cells and decrease moisture loss, while also helping to destroy free radicals, the oxidizing agents that age the skin. However, they are both expensive oils

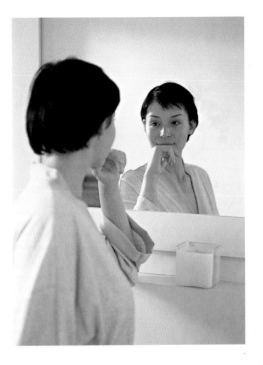

so are normally blended with one of the above, roughly in a proportion of one part to every seven of the main oil. They benefit all skin types.

Like wheatgerm, however, evening primrose and borage oil are inclined to go rancid. To prevent this happening, add vitamin E, which is an antioxidant. You can buy capsules of vitamin E oil, which you simply break open and drip into the base oil when you first open the bottle. The vitamin E will be used up as it absorbs and destroys the free radicals, so you will need to add more if you keep these oils for any period of time.

flower power

As natural substances, oils have distinctive and not universally appealing aromas. So ever since the ancient Greeks put marjoram and mint in their skin oils, people have perfumed them.

The simplest, safest and most beneficial way to perfume a vegetable or nut oil is undoubtedly to use essential oils. Many commercial skin preparations now contain – and highly publicize – essential oil, but at least 90 per cent of what you smell will be made from synthetic chemicals. Several hundred raw ingredients can be used to create a single artificial fragrance and they are the second most common cause of allergy, sensitization or irritation in commercial cosmetics. Neither do they have the therapeutic benefits of essential oils.

What are essential oils?

An essential oil is a concentrated, aromatic, volatile liquid made up of tiny oil-like molecules that blend easily with vegetable or nut oil. They do not contain any fatty substances, so do not stain.

The 'oil' comes from the small cavities in the cellular structure of plants or peel of fruits and is extracted by distillation or cold pressing, which concentrates them into powerful substances: it takes 100 kg of rose petals to produce 20 ml of rose oil, for example. So, while natural, they are strong enough to sensitize the skin or even cause allergic reactions. But this is far less likely than with the synthetic fragrances used in commercial skin products. Their potency means you use them in a very dilute form. If mixed with a carrier oil, a dilution of 1–2 per cent is enough; in a bath, 5–8 drops.

How can they help?

Essential oils effect their magic in four ways:
1. They penetrate the dermis. They are able to do this because they are made up of tiny molecules and are lipophilic (attracted to fats). So they pass through the hair follicles, which contain sebum, and from there they are absorbed into the bloodstream or lymph system.
2. They do not create a dependency or stop the skin reacting, as it does when it gets used to some products.
3. They all repel infection and boost circulation.
4. Many also stimulate new cell growth, which is particularly important if you are the 'wrong' side of 30.

However, if essential oils oxidize, they lose their therapeutic properties. To maximize their shelf life, keep them in a cool, dark place and do not leave them unopened. They should last at least a year. Mixing with a carrier oil drastically reduces their lifespan to two or three months.

Their effects are not only directly physical. They also act via the nasal tract to affect the pleasure pathways in the brain. So it is no good choosing an essential oil for its purported anti-ageing properties alone. You also have to like the smell. That said, those on the table opposite are worth a sniff.

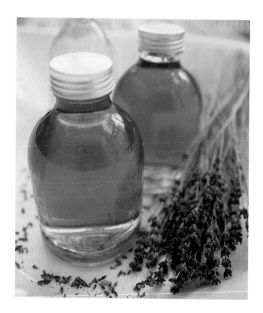

Oil	Skin type	Properties	Blends well with	Carrier oils	Contraindications
Frankincense	Ageing	Tones and firms	Geranium, lavender	Apricot, almond	
Lavender	All types, including dry, ageing and damaged	Aids regeneration of damaged skin, calms inflammation	Palmarosa, geranium, rosewood	Macadamia, light olive, calendula, almond	
Neroli	Dry, ageing	Firms, aids cell regeneration, helps with thread veins, stretch marks and scars	Geranium, lavender	Avocado, hazelnut, apricot	Not for very sensitive skins
Fennel	Ageing	Contains easily absorbed oestrogen-like molecules that may help with wrinkles	Frankincense, lavender, neroli	Avocado, madadamia, evening primrose	Avoid in pregnancy
Geranium	Dry, ageing and normal, puffy	Tones, firms, stimulates bloodflow	Lavender, bergamot	Soya, apricot	Increases sensitivity to UV rays
Bergamot	Normal to oily	Calms and helps prevent inflammation, limits bacterial growth. Good for infected skin	Geranium, ylang ylang	Safflower, almond, sunflower	
Rosewood	All types	Limits bacterial growth, soothes, firms, stimulates cell growth, aids circulation	Lavender, neroli, geranium	Jojoba, soya, hazelnut	
Patchouli	Ageing, damaged, combination	Firms, increases circulation, calms inflammation, good for chapped and cracked skin	Geranium, palmarosa, rose otto	Jojoba, macadamia, hazelnut	
Sandalwood	Normal-to-dry	Destroys bacteria, soothes dry, sensitive and irritated skins	Geranium, palmarosa, bergamot	Avocado, almond, calendula	Not for sensitive or irritated skin
Myrrh	Ageing, damaged	Anti-inflammatory, antiseptic, heals open spots and blemishes	Cypress, frankincense, geranium, tea tree	Jojoba, almond	Avoid in pregnancy
Rose otto	Dry, ageing, damaged or sensitive	Stimulates, balances, limits bacterial growth, strengthens fragile capillaries	Clary sage, lavender, cypress	Hazelnut, borage, lime blossom	
Palmarosa	Dry-to-normal, ageing	Regenerative, good for wrinkles and scars	Geranium, rosewood, sandalwood	Avocado, hazelnut, lime blossom	
Tea tree	Normal-to-oil	Repels and destroys bacteria, good for acne and fungal growth	Lavender, ylang ylang	Jojoba, macadamia	
Cypress	Oily or open-pored, congested, reddened or puffy	Aids blood and lymphatic flow, helps with thread veins	Geranium, ylang ylang	Hazelnut, borage, calendula	Avoid in early pregnancy
Lemon	Oily or infected	Firms, limits bacterial growth, removes dead cells, increases circulation	Ylang ylang, rose otto	Hazelnut, thistle	Increases reaction to sunlight. Irritation on sensitive skin
Ylang ylang	Oily and combination	Firms, moderates sebum production	Palmarosa, lavender, cypress	Thistle, sunflower	
Roman Chamomile	Damaged, oily, ageing	Calms inflammation and bacterial infection. Good for dry, sensitive skin and thread veins	Rosewood, lavender, sandalwood	Olive, calendula, hazelnut	Avoid in early pregnancy

four-minute massage

You can do this after removing make-up using a carrier oil or while applying your moisturizing cream. Once you have memorized the routine it should take no more than 3–4 minutes. So try to do it every day.

1. Pour just under a teaspoon of oil into one hand, rub it into both and apply the oil to your neck and face in long, upward and outward sweeping movements. Apply it very sparingly around your eyes, where the skin is most delicate, using the ring finger of both hands.

2. Using your hands alternately, slide up your neck from the base to your jaw bone, turning the hands as necessary and working lightly over your windpipe. Cover your whole neck from ear to ear.

3. Using the index and middle fingers of each hand, slide firmly along your jaw line from your chin to the front of your ears. Your index finger should be on top of your jaw and the middle finger underneath.

4. With your fingers together and hands pointing up to your brow, holding the fingers straight, press firmly with the edge of your hands either side of your nose. Hold for 3–4 seconds.

5. Release the pressure slightly and, rolling your hands on to your cheeks, slide your hands outwards with your index fingers stopping in front of your ears and apply a firm pressure. Hold for 3–4 seconds. Repeat.

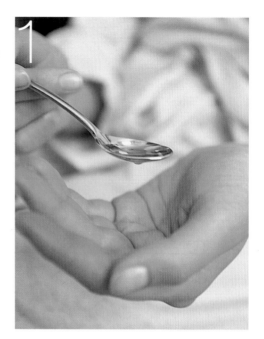

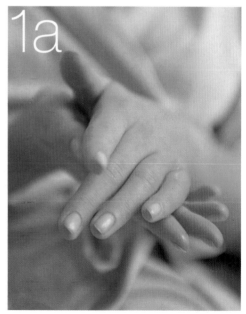

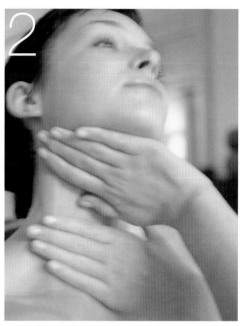

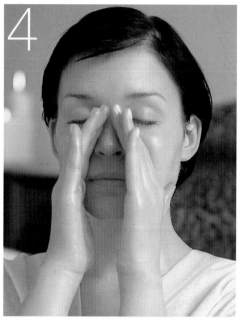

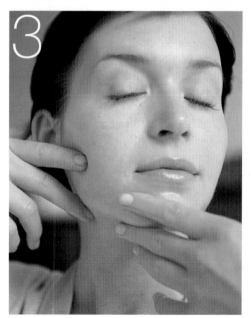

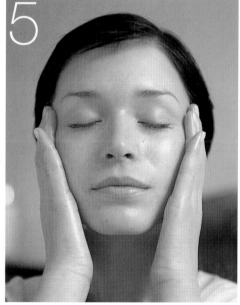

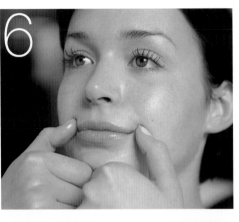

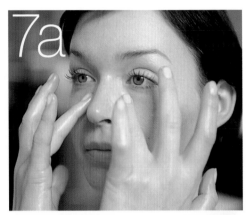

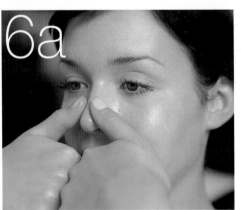

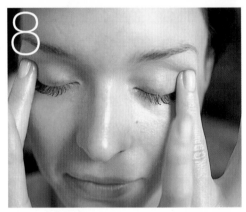

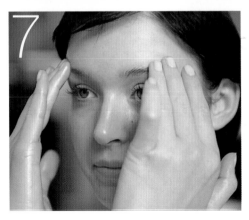

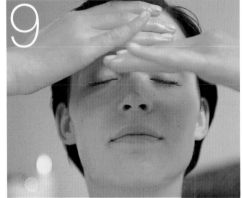

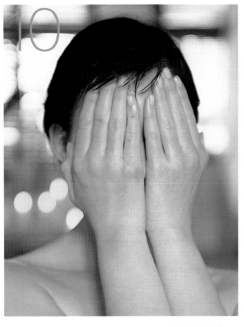

6. With your fingers held underneath your chin, slide both thumbs upwards symmetrically around the corners of your mouth, in under your nose, around your nostrils and lightly off over the tip of your nose.

7. With the middle and ring fingers of each hand, starting at the inner corners of your eyebrows, slide firmly outwards over your eyebrows and, using your ring finger only, trace very lightly inwards underneath your eyes.

8. With the ring finger of each hand, slide lightly outwards over your closed eyelids and then lightly underneath each eye.

9. With your fingers together and the index fingers leading the way, smooth the palms of the hands one after the other up to the hairline in a firm lifting movement, starting between the eyebrows and finishing at the hairline.

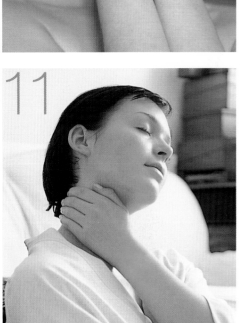

10. Close your eyes and, with the fingers together and using the whole of both hands slightly cupped to produce a gentle suction, apply a firm pressure to the face, holding for a second before releasing. Then, moving the hands outwards from the nose towards the ears, cover the whole face, moving the hands up and down to cover the area between the chin and hairline.

11. With your fingers together and using the whole of the hand, apply pressure with the right hand to the left side of the neck, working from the base of the neck to the jaw but avoiding the windpipe. Repeat with the left hand, applying pressures to the right side of the neck.

fifteen-minute massage

An extended version of the 4-minute massage, best done at the end of the day.

1. Pour about two teaspoons of oil into one hand, rub it into both and apply the oil to your face, neck, shoulders and upper arms.

2. Using the knuckes of both hands pointing inwards, make circular kneading movements all over the upper chest.

3. Using the hands alternately, knuckle over the upper arms (deltoids) and upper shoulder muscles (trapezius). Make sure the arm being worked on is as relaxed as possible.

4. One hand at a time, with flat fingertips make a kneading, squeezing movement over the top of the opposite shoulder to the large trapezius muscle that helps support the head. While working on the shoulders, support the working arm at the elbow.

5. Using both hands, with the flat fingertips of the middle three fingers, apply firm, circular pressures on the muscles either side of the spine from the base of the skull to the base of the neck.

6. Working with one hand at a time on the opposite shoulder, with flat fingertips apply slow, deep pressures into the muscle on top of the shoulders, behind the collar-bone. Start at the end of the muscle just inside the shoulder and work gradually inwards towards the base of the neck. Press firmly and deeply, increasing gently where it feels tender and holding until the tension seems to release.

Follow step 2 from the 4-minute massage (see pages 36–37).

7. With the fingers of one hand, apply gentle pressure by the side of and slightly under the Adam's apple for 7–10 seconds. Repeat on both sides twice, using alternate hands.

Follow step 3 from the 4-minute massage.

8. With flat fingertips slightly spaced out, apply firm pressures along the top of the jaw bone from the chin outwards and towards the angle of the jaw. Then move up to the cheeks, applying firm pressures in rows upwards over the cheeks. Repeat, making each row slightly higher up the face, with the last row finishing on top of the cheekbones.

9. Use the pads of the index and middle fingers in circular pressures to massage the joint of the jaw bone that stands out when you clench your teeth.

Follow step 4 from the 4-minute massage.

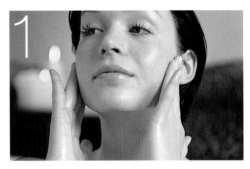

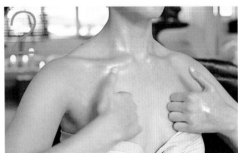

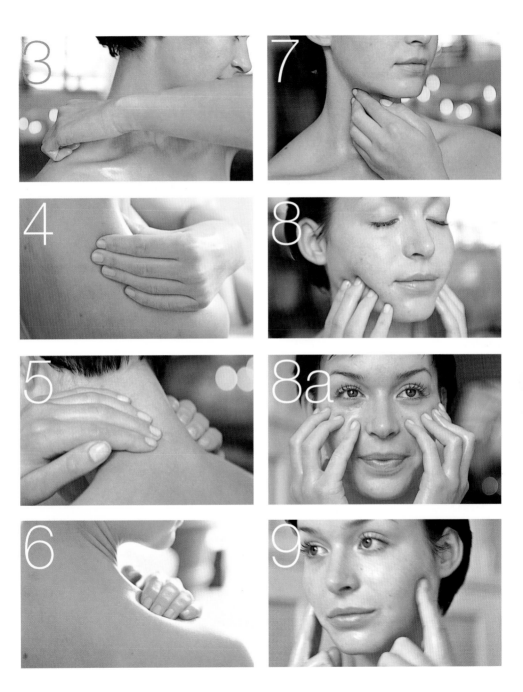

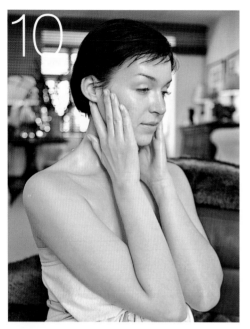

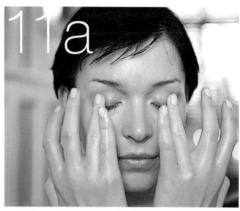

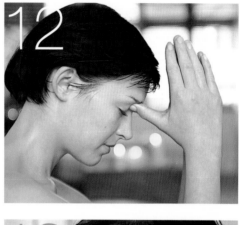

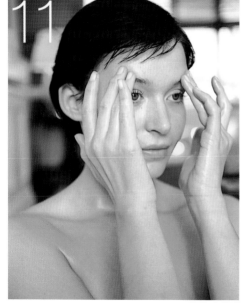

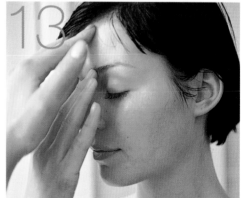

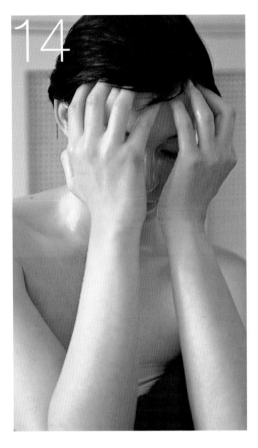

10. Place your hands on the sides of the face and position the index fingers behind the ears and the other fingers in front. Apply pressures, moving downwards from in front of the ears towards the angle of the jaw.

Follow steps 6, 7 and 8 from the 4-minute massage.

11. With the pads of the index and middle fingers of each hand, apply firm pressure, moving the hands outwards along the line of the eyebrows and then with your ring fingers inwards underneath the eyes, pressing along the sockets.

12. Resting your elbows on the table, press firmly with your thumbs above the inner corner of the eyes, relaxing your head on to your thumbs. The point is often sensitive, so start the pressure gently, increasing gradually as the tension is relieved. Apply pressures all along the upper ridge of the eye socket.

13. Using the hands alternately, with the index and middle finger of each hand apply a firm pressure on the inner corners of your eyebrows. Release slightly and slide straight up from your forehead to the hairline. Repeat in a flowing, continuous movement five to six times.

Follow steps 9, 10 and 11 from the 4-minute routine.

14. Using both hands together and with the fingertips slightly spaced, use the fingerpads to apply rows of firm pressures from the eyebrows upwards towards the hairline, covering the whole of the forehead.

problem areas

You may have areas of your face that are calling for extra attention. The exercises below work for remedial or preventive purposes, and can be fitted into the 4-minute or the 15-minute massage routine.

1. For a double chin

With the fingers relaxed, use the thumbs to press into the muscle underneath the jaw, starting in the centre of the chin and working outwards towards the angle of the jaw bone.

This can be done after step 2 in the 4-minute massage or after step 6 in the 15-minute massage.

2. For jowls

Using the flat middle and ring fingers of both hands alternately and treating one side at a time, work on the muscles of the cheeks (the masseter and zygomaticus: see diagram on page 53) with a rolling, lifting movement, almost flicking the muscle upwards.

Do after step 4 in the 4-minute massage or after step 10 in the 15-minute massage.

3–4. For wrinkled lips

Smiling to stretch the lips taut, and anchoring the middle finger of your left hand on the left corner of the mouth, use the middle finger of the right hand to make small, circular movements all the way along the edge of the bottom lip. Then swap hands to use the middle finger of the left hand and repeat the circles on the edge of the upper lip.

Do after step 6 in the 4-minute massage or after step 10 in the 15-minute massage.

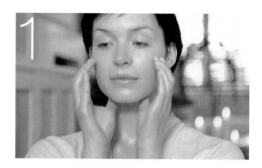

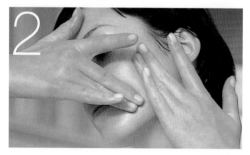

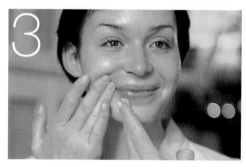

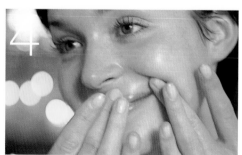

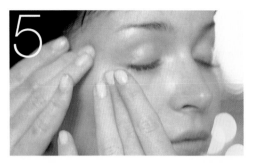

5. For crow's feet

With the middle or ring finger of each hand, make a crossroads shape where the crow's feet are emerging by tracing a horizontal then a vertical line, alternately working with the middle fingers of each hand, out from the corner of your eye and up towards the temple.

Do after step 8 in the 4-minute massage or step 10 in the 15-minute massage.

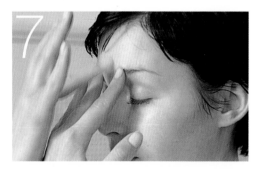

6. For open pores on the nose and between the eyes

With your middle or ring finger, make small circular movements all over and around your nose. Start by working around your nostrils, over the tip of your nose and up the sides of your nose, finishing on the bridge of the nose.

Do after step 2 in the 4-minute massage or step 6 in the 15-minute massage.

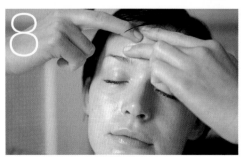

7. For frown lines between the eyes

With the index and middle fingers of your left hand supporting the skin in an upward 'V' shape, apply small circular movements with the ring finger of your right hand between the eyebrows. Do this after step 8 in the 4-minute massage or step 12 in the 15-minute massage.

8. For brow lines on the forehead

Locate the brow lines across your forehead. Starting above your right eye, make small, circular, sliding movements along each line from right to left using the middle finger of your right hand. Use the index and middle fingers of your left hand to hold the skin firm on either side of the line. Repeat the movement on each line. Do after step 9 in the 4-minute massage or step 14 in the 15-minute massage.

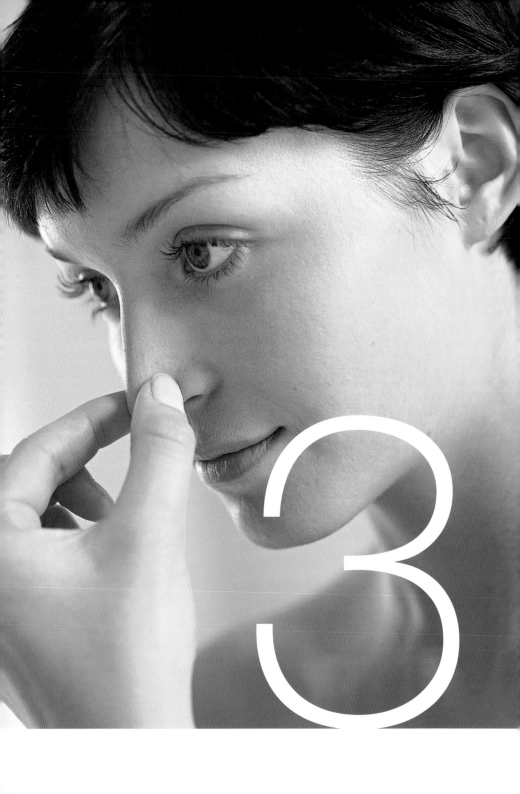

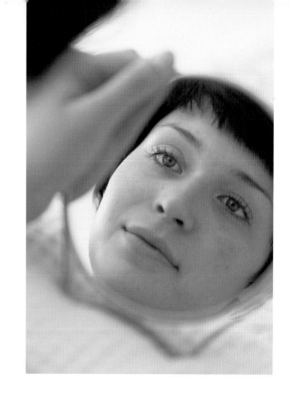

keep
your face fit

voluntary work

Walk into any gym and you see people exercising their muscles until the sweat runs freely. The biceps, triceps and quadraceps are all being forced through their paces in an effort to build and tone them, all the better to cope with the demands of daily life.

The vogue for aerobic exercise and body sculpting that dominated the 1980s and 1990s has made even the most stubbornly sedentary people more aware of the importance of muscle tone to their general health and appearance.

Hard work?

But in the average day, which of the 656 muscles in the body work the longest hours and get noticed most? Undoubtedly the 50-plus in the face – not that their owners notice. You cannot help being conscious of sagging stomach muscles or droopy buttocks because you are always having to tuck them into trousers or hide them under dresses. The face muscles just sit there until called upon, invariably out of sight and out of mind.

All muscles in the body are crudely divided into voluntary and involuntary ones. Those upon which life depends are the involuntary ones – which is just as well, or in the clutter of everyday life we might forget to breathe!

The muscles controlling the face, like those directing the limbs, are clearly voluntary. But the big difference from other such muscles is that the facial ones are more often than not used unconsciously. Night and day, they undergo a punishing regime. When you are dreaming, your eyelids are moving or your jaw is grinding your teeth. As you are reading this, you may well be frowning (stop it!). When you are talking on the phone, though no one can see it, your face will be expressing your words.

So the face is constantly being exercised. The problem is that it is often a negative kind of exercise, because the muscles are being tensed and stretched in unequal measures at different times.

Team work

Muscles are designed to work in small teams and to be complementary. So one muscle raises the forehead while another lowers it, one curls your lower lip while another pulls it back. When used for the purposes for which they were ideally designed, they work in harmony, with one contracting when its team-mate stretches.

But unconscious, habitual expressions often distort that harmonious pattern, causing certain muscles to be overstretched or unduly contracted while their partners suffer the reverse misfortune. And what happens in any tissues that are unequally stretched, relaxed or contracted? Corrugations form deep in their structure – and these soon rise to the surface as wrinkles.

Furthermore, if both sides of the face are not consciously exercised in equal measure, as they were designed to be, they become asymmetrical – and symmetry, as many studies in nature have shown, is a fundamental principle of beauty. Lop-sided contours and wrinkles emerge all over the body eventually. But they tend to occur more quickly in the face because of the way in which all but one of its muscles are attached at one end to tissue rather than bone.

Since the face is evidently made up of muscle, skin, tissue and nerves like any other part of the anatomy, why does it not occur to even the most self-conscious individuals to keep it exercised and toned? Partly because the unremitting claims and promises of the beauty industry convince people that the only solution to lines and wrinkles in the face is an external one, but also because people are not routinely aware of the muscles of their face, however hard they may make them work on a daily basis.

The first trick, then, is to become as aware of the facial muscles as you are of other voluntary muscles in the body.

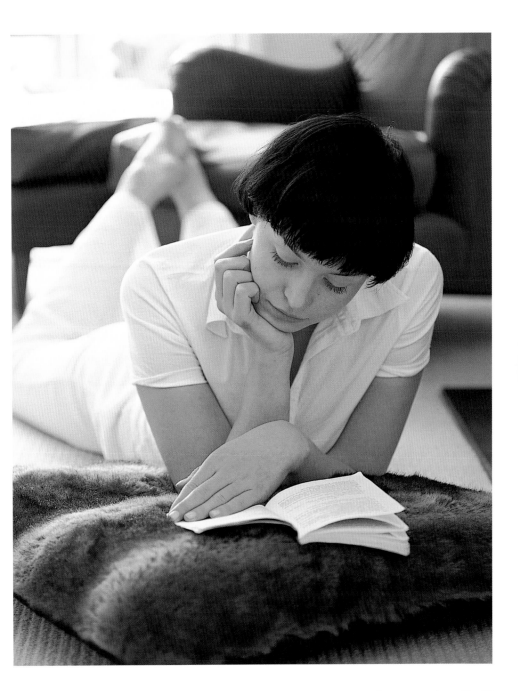

muscles that matter

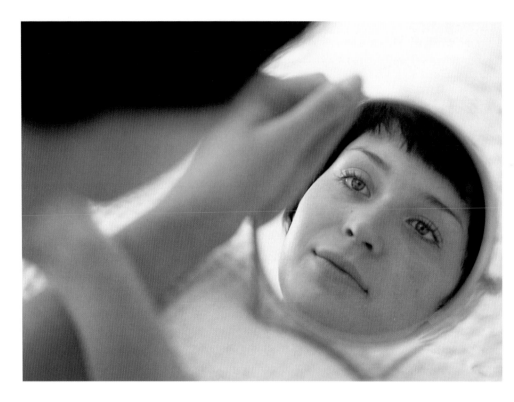

You need to learn to regard the facial muscles in much the same way as the panting figure doing sit-ups in the gym does the rectus abdominalis that hold in his or her stomach like a girdle.

Facial exercise

The facial muscles influence one's contours just as much and, most importantly, are just as easily trained. Of course, the shape of your face is fundamentally determined by your bone structure. You can do little about the bulbous Roman nose or obtrusive ears you have inherited, without the help of a cosmetic surgeon. However, you can make your chin stronger, your eyes less hollow, your lips fuller or your cheeks more prominent by exercising the muscles there.

The muscles responsible for facial expression are in two or even three layers, most with one end anchored to the bone and the other to a sheath of connective tissue. Exercise helps you to feel these muscles working and so to be aware when they are 'exercising' themselves to ill-effect. More often than we might like to think, our facial muscles are used to form grimaces, twitches and scowls – the very movements that pull the face down. As we have seen, where muscles go, the skin to which they are attached eventually follows.

A fact oft quoted but worth repeating is that it takes twice as much muscular effort to frown as to smile. Smiling involves only the zygomatic major muscle, but to frown you need to contract two or even three muscles.

All muscles degenerate with age. The resulting facial sag starts very subtly and slowly in one's twenties, becomes noticeable in one's thirties and invariably turns into a preoccupation by one's forties. But equal and upward exercise will always bulk them out and raise them up, even if the speed and efficacy with which they can be built up declines gradually as the years roll by.

Bottoms up

If you are still not convinced that the condition of the facial muscles defines your face just as the rower's deltoids and pectorals define their shoulders and chest, try this. Put a mirror on the floor and stand with your back to it. Now spread your feet apart so that you are firmly balanced. Bending from the hips, hang your head right down so that you are looking at your upside-down face. See the loose folds of skin? More muscle, as you probably once had, would help take up that slack.

Now what you need to do is make yourself aware of your facial muscles when you are not looking upside-down in a mirror.

If you have started to massage, you are already learning where they are and how they feel externally. Exercise helps you to feel them work as individual items. You cannot expect to be ever-conscious of all of them. But if you learn to control the 18 main muscles (see page 53), you can begin to rejuvenate your whole face.

Feeling your face

While the muscles of the face are among the body's busiest, they are by no means the easiest to control. Tell anyone to sprint along a track and, stamina permitting, they can do it. Ask them to lift a hefty dumb-bell and, as long as they keep their balance, they will at least know how. But many people cannot flare their nostrils, move their ears or shift their scalp.

This is because the muscles that control such movements are not those we need to call on in the daily run of things. Fortunately, neither do those particular ones affect the shape or tone of the face, so they are not integral to an exercise routine. But there are other underused facial muscles over which you need to gain control.

These muscles are not completely dormant. You may often move them in your sleep or involuntarily when you flex other, more major muscles. But how do you learn to feel them and to move them consciously? It is a bit like learning to speak a foreign language. You have to learn which muscles produce which movements. One reason that immigrants and émigrés invariably keep their strong accents is that they continue to use the same muscles and movements in their tongue, throat and lips as they did in their own language to try to produce the new sounds.

This will never work. They need first to find out, from someone who does it naturally, the position their tongue should be in to produce the sound and then persistently try the sound in isolation. Nine times out of ten it will eventually come out spontaneously.

Physical persistence is only one side of the equation; imagination is the other. Visualizing the muscles you need to exercise, but cannot quite feel, can help to bring them into conscious play.

age is no excuse

The younger you start facial gymnastics, the better. If you begin in your twenties, you can postpone the wrinkles by several years. Younger muscles are built up more quickly through exercise than older ones and, because they are more elastic, are less susceptible to damage.

But by the same token, it is never too late. In fact, exercises are recommended for people who have had cosmetic surgery on their faces – most of that group being in their late forties and early fifties. Some enlightened surgeons now recommend that patients start on a facial exercise programme before they have surgery, to strengthen the muscle and makes it more resilient during the recovery period and easier to continue building up afterwards.

How a muscle ages

From one's early thirties, muscle all over the body starts to shrink as its fibres lose protein. While the number of fibres remains the same, their diameter decreases, so muscle thins out. Muscle also gets drier, and so loses fluid bulk. But it does not lose length, and may even become longer as a result of being stretched. This is what gives rise to the droopy look seen in old age.

The process is slow and imperceptible – until you compare a picture of someone's upper arms at 25 and 45. The muscles on the upper body atrophy more quickly because they are not forced to carry weight every day. Considering the effect on the arms, which we do use for lifting if not continual weight-bearing like the legs, imagine how much more quickly the facial muscles must shrink.

Another consequence of muscle shrinkage is that it is accompanied by a drop in the production of steroid hormones from the adrenal and sex glands. These hormones are responsible for, among other things, smooth, supple skin. Exercise can help slow down the decline in hormone levels. So keeping the muscles active has multiple benefits.

Supplementary benefits

The muscles under the skin are not the only things to benefit from exercise. A facial work-out also seems to have an effect on the adjoining connective tissue. By increasing the supply of oxygen and nutrients to the tissue, exercise is thought to stimulate cell growth in the elastic fibres within collagen and elastin that naturally atrophy with age.

Another diminishing asset on the ageing face is fat. Although most women spend years regarding adipose tissue as their worst enemy, when it disappears from their face they miss it. For in the space where fat once sat, wrinkles congregate. This is most noticeable where the skin is thinnest, such as around the eyes. When that area loses some of its fatty tissue, the eyes take on a hollow look, often exaggerated by circles of darkening skin. As fat stores atrophy all over the face, it gets more gaunt .

One option is to up the calorie count, put in a regular order at the chip shop and accept wobbly hips. A more attractive solution is to fill the skin out again with muscle through exercise.

The muscles of the face

There are more than 50 muscles in the face itself (see diagram, right) and more than 40 others that contribute to facial movements, most of these being in the neck and upper shoulders. But don't worry – you have to exercise fewer than half of them to make a big difference to the tone and contours of your face.

1 Temporalis the muscles of the temple which enable the jaw to close

2 Frontalis the muscles of the forehead which are responsible for the furrowing of the brow

3 Orbucularis oculi the ring muscle around the eye is responsible for the lines associated with laughing and smiling

4 Quadratus labii superioris the upper lip muscle conjures a smile on the upper lip

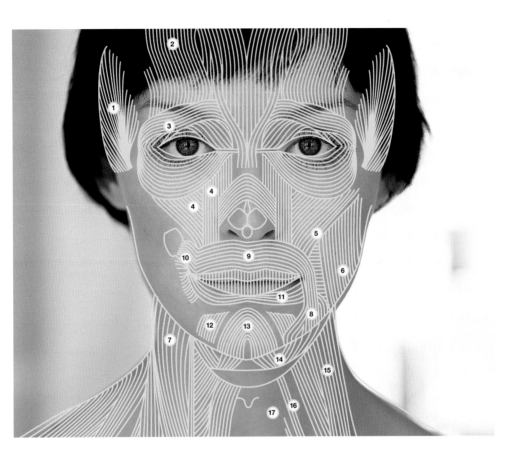

5 Zygomaticus the cheekbone muscle that helps to move the mouth

6 Masseter the chewing muscle that closes the jaw

7 Sterno-cleido-mastoideus this muscle connects the chest and collar bone to the skull and allows the head to be turned

8 Triangularis the drooping of the corners of the mouth in states of displeasure, is facilitated by this triangular muscle

9 Orbucularis the upper ring muscle of the lip is also responsible for the movement of the lips

10 Buccinator these deep cheek muscles are responsible for the formation of dimples

11 Orbicularis orbis inferioris the lower lip ring muscle is also able to move the lips

12 Quadratis labii inferioris the lower quadreatic lip muscle

13 Mentalis the chin muscle

14 Digastricus this muscle is responsible for holding in the 'double chin' and keeps the lower jaw flexible

15 Scalenus medius the uneven-sided triangular muscle

16 Omhyoideus the shoulderblade muscle

17 Sternohyoideus this is the breastbone-hyoid-bone muscle

posture

The sedentary lifestyles that most of us have these days do our faces no favours. Used to slumping and slouching, we usually only sit up and take notice when backache or shoulder strain forces us to do so. But bad posture has equally negative effects on the face and neck. Holding the body upright is a form of exercise that conditions the neck and face muscles. If the muscles in the shoulders and neck are weakened or twisted by bad posture, the resulting tension will reduce blood flow to the face.

Posture is affected by many parts of the body. But if you concentrate on the four major areas outlined below, you can make a big enough difference to see it reflected in your face.

Neck

Human babies learn to walk far later than other mammals because, to house their larger brains, they need disproportionately large heads. By adulthood the proportion may have equalled out but the head, at around five kilos, still requires the full support of the neck to hold it up. Most people hold their heads too far back, putting a big strain on the neck to pull it forward – in effect so that the weight of the head will not pull you over backwards! The resulting tension in the neck interrupts blood flow to the face and deprives the supporting muscles of the exercise they need, so they lose muscle. The most obvious consequence is a wrinkly neck. Since the neck tends to age earlier than the face anyway, this is a problem you don't need.

To release tension in the neck, do some daily neck bends. Breathing out, relax the shoulders and drop the head forward. Then rock it back to rest on the top of the spine and sideways towards each shoulder. Do not worry if you hear and feel alarming creaks at every point. This happens as the knots of tension are released.

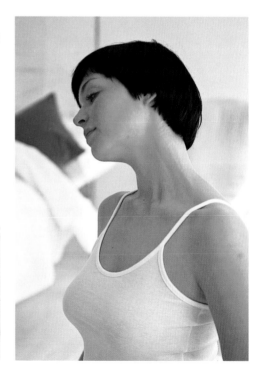

To help hold the neck as the extension of the spine that it should be, try this visualization. When you are sitting or walking about during the daily run of things imagine that a string extends upwards from the crown of your head, pulling it skyward. This visualization should help you hold your head upright at the crucial joint where the skull meets the first vertebra.

Alternatively, imagine your head to be a balloon that is pulling the top of you up slightly. At the same time, do try not to hunch your shoulders but keep them broad and relaxed and pulled down away from your ears.

Upper back and shoulders

When people are reminded of their bad posture, the first thing they do is pull their shoulders back as if on military parade. But this creates tension in the neck and shoulders, shortens the spine and restricts breathing. Instead, keep your back broad and think of your spine extending so that the space between each vertebra increases.

Imagine your shoulder-blades, comfortably apart, dropping down always from your ears and towards your buttocks. This opens up the rib cage, enabling the back muscles to lengthen, and gives the lungs plenty of room to expand.

Pelvis

The pelvis marks the centre of gravity in the body, so is crucial to good posture. You only need to look at the smooth gait of a professional dancer, who characteristically glides along from the hips, to see that it is central to good balance.

What the rest of us do is unconsciously to drop it forward, which not only puts a strain on the lower back but makes the bottom ungraciously stick out. To correct this, do some daily pelvic thrusts. Think Elvis Presley or Michael Jackson and shoot the pelvis forward repeatedly.

Feet

There is perhaps no part of a woman's body more routinely neglected or abused than her feet. In the name of fashion, they get shoved into shoes of a shape that bear as much relation to a human foot as a pumpkin to a banana skin. The resulting bunions, blisters and calluses may keep chiropodists in business, but they do nothing for your posture. What is more, the first place in which discomfort visibly registers is in your face.

In bare feet or wearing soft shoes, stand with your feet flat on the floor shoulder-width apart. Spread the weight equally between the heels and balls of your feet and your slightly-spread toes.

Do not rest more on one foot than the other as the imbalance transfers itself to one hip or the other and from there to the spine, which then twists to compensate, making the neck tense.

Take your time

Just as a muscle ages slowly, so it improves slowly with exercise. Don't be tempted to do more than indicated in order to achieve quicker results: you won't, and the relentless effort will probably make you give up and go in search of the latest 'once-a-day rejuvenating gel'.

In the short term, you should see an improvement in your complexion within minutes of exercising. But this is due to the increase in blood circulation and lymph flow rather than a firmer muscle. You could get the same effect standing on your head every morning for a few minutes. The effect may last a day but will wane if you do not exercise at least every other day.

Because they vary in size and their proximity to the surface skin, muscles seem to improve at different rates. The improvement in the tone of your cheeks, for example, should be visible within a few weeks. However results in the neck and jaw may take longer to show.

three steps to a fit face

All the exercises in the routines below and over the next few pages follow a similar three-part pattern, based on the following common principles:

Finding Obvious though it may seem that before exercising a muscle you need to find it, doing so is not automatic. Dormant muscles will be less than prominent and small ones may take practice to locate. At first, it will help if you look in the mirror while doing the exercise. (If this makes you laugh, all the better: crow's feet are preferable to furrows on your forehead.)

Resisting Providing resistance against which the muscle can exert its force limits the blood flow to the muscle. The flow is then increased and the oxygen in the new rush of blood feeds and builds up the muscle.

Relaxing The exercised muscle needs to be consciously relaxed after it has been tensed. Otherwise, the tension and tightness will interfere with good blood circulation and may produce muscle cramps.

Tips for facial exercise

• Always make sure your face is relaxed before you start (see page 117).
• Apply a light cream or oil, which helps to minimize any stretching of the skin. Ensure your face is clean before you put on any lubricant.
• Warm up the muscles before you begin to exercise them, particularly if you are exercising a 'problem area' regularly.
• While you are getting used to these exercises, place a mirror at head height so that you can comfortably follow the moves and watch your face as you exercise.

• Never pull the skin: in resistance exercises, it is the muscle that must be moved, not the skin.
• If you feel any pain, stop. It probably means you are using the wrong muscles. Read the instructions, try to visualize the muscles, concentrate on them and attempt the exercise again later.
• In exercises for muscles that mirror each other on either side of your face, exercise each side equally. Symmetry is one of the fundamental principles of bodily beauty.
• Exercise every day if possible: as with other forms of bodily toning, a little regularly is more effective than a bumper session once in a while.
• Take time over each exercise: there is more benefit in doing one exercise properly than ten in passing.
• Relax between exercises. The relaxation period should be as long as each exercise period.
• Focus on your breathing and do not hold your breath in or out.
• Even if you feel tired or in a hurry, follow the 'cool-down' routine afterwards.

Although few of us have the time every day to ensure that all these conditions are met before we commit ourselves to start, in contrast with exercises for other parts of the body facial exercises require no special gear, garments or venues. You can do them virtually anytime, anywhere: in queues; at your desk; and in the bathroom.

Although you may get some strange looks, when bemused or amused onlookers find themselves with descending jowls and deepening crow's feet, you will be having the last laugh.

Before and after

When training any part of the body through exercise, it is important to warm up and cool down. A warm-up helps to relieve any tension in the muscles and to increase circulation, while a quick cool-down routine helps to prevent cramp or aches developing. The face is no exception and will benefit most from the exercises on the following pages if warmed-up and cooled-down.

Warm-up Either standing or sitting upright, extend the arms out to the sides at shoulder height. Make ten small circular movements forwards with the whole arm, rotating from the shoulder sockets. Do the same moving the arms backwards. Repeat three to five times each way, increasing the size of the circles with each repetition. This helps to loosen up the whole throat and neck area, improving blood flow.

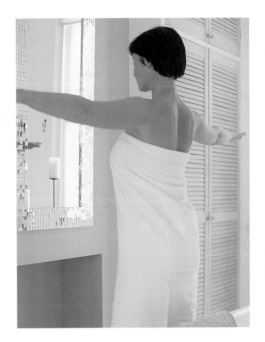

Cool-down Repeat the procedure for the warm-up, then slump down forwards with your head almost touching your knees. The whole upper body should be limp, with the arms hanging like pendulums. Breathe in and out deeply.

   This helps to keep up the flow of lymph, which drains away any toxins that may have built up during your exercise routine.

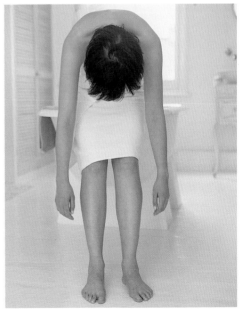

exercise routines

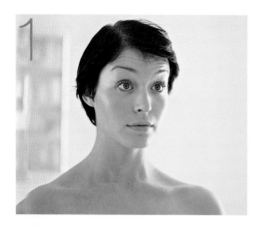

You don't need to do all of these exercises. Simply choose four or five of them that work on the areas you want to improve and spend no more than a minute on each. Starting with a bookstand and mirror at home, practicse the moves until you can relinquish the promts and props and exercise on the move, grabbing five minutes whenever and wherever you can.

Forehead

Works on the frontalis muscle that runs across the brow. Helps prevent or lessen horizontal frown lines.

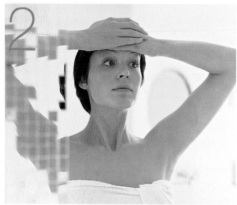

1. The frontalis muscle is easy to identify: simply raise your brow.

2. Lay your hands on top of each other on your forehead with the fingertips pointing inward and press. Don't be afraid to press firmly as this is the one facial muscle that is attached to two bones. Now raise the muscle up towards your scalp against the pressure of your hands. Hold for five seconds, then rest. Repeat four times.

3. To relax the brow muscle, just close the eyes and look cross-eyed for 5–10 seconds. Repeat 3–4 times.

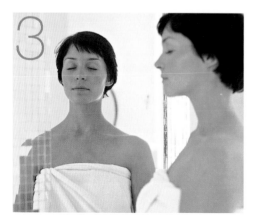

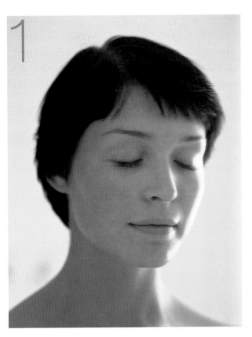

Eyes

Works on the eye ring muscle. Helps to raise droopy eyelids and to postpone the emergence, and lessen the severity, of crow's feet.

1. Close your eyes and stare strongly. What you feel is the orbucularis oculi – the circular ring of muscle that runs around each eye.

2. With your eyes still shut, tighten them, screwing them up and directing the pupils inward, cross-eyed. Hold for a few seconds. Open your eyes as wide as possible and immediately stare at a fixed point so that the pupil is centred.

3. Blink rapidly and repeatedly 10–15 times, opening your eyes wide each time, then gently close them again. Wait until the pupils feel as if they have returned to normal.

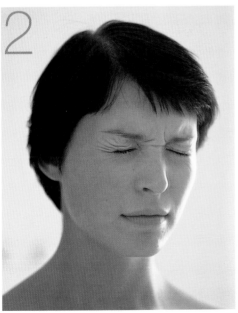

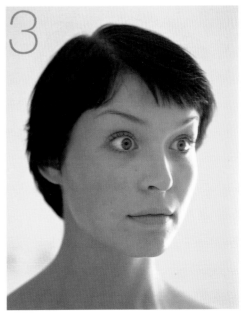

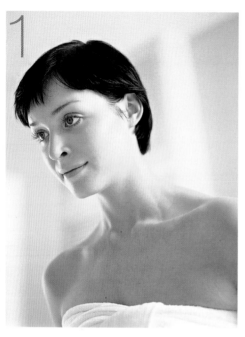

Nose

Works on the musculus vasalis, the main muscle in the nose, which is connected to the bone in which the eye teeth are anchored. Helps to prevent enlargement of the nose (which grows with age) by firming the muscle and keeping it flexible.

1. Puff up both nostrils as you breathe in slowly and strongly. Draw your nose up and sniff. Contract the nostrils while breathing out. Repeat 6–7 times.

2. Repeat as above, while holding your nostrils gently between your thumb and index finger. Slowly breathe out through your nose, feeling your chest sink downwards.

3. With your index finger, push the tip of your nose up then pull it down between your thumb and index finger. Repeat 4–5 times.

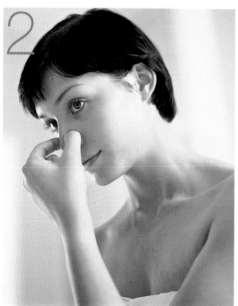

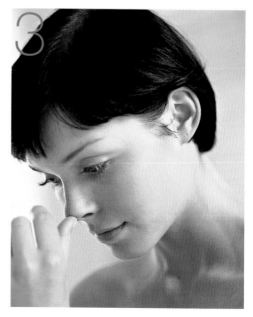

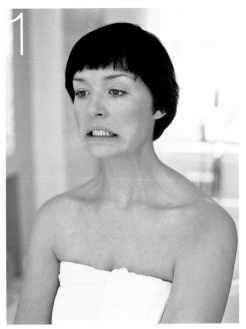

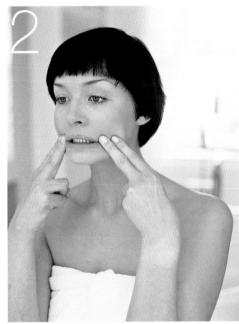

Mouth and Chin

Works on the lower quadratic lip muscle that moves the bottom lip and on the small triangular chin muscle. Helps to prevent the corners of the mouth and the chin drooping and to raise emerging jowls. Also improves the contour and tone of the lips.

1. Open your lips while keeping your upper and lower teeth together. Then pull the corners of your mouth sideways so that the bottom row of teeth becomes visible.

2. Press your index fingers into the two corners of your mouth and, using the muscles, pull the corners down against the resistance of your fingers.

3. Open your mouth slightly and lightly shake your head to loosen tension around your chin.

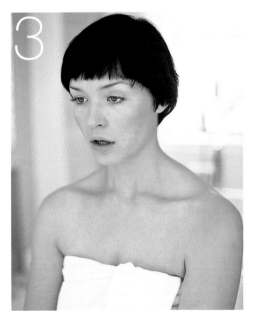

exercises for problem areas

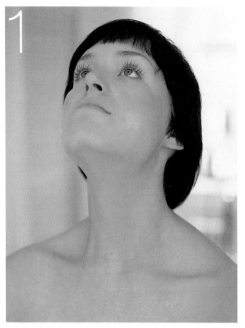

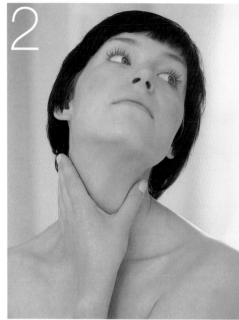

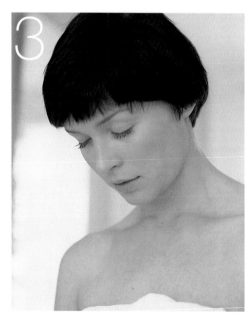

Neck

Works on the four main muscles that run down the
neck on either side of the Adam's apple. Helps to
firm up the throat and lift the breast tissue, while
increasing circulation to the whole face.

1. Tip your head back and jut out your bottom jaw.
Pushing your chin forward so that the lower teeth
overlap the upper ones, feel your neck muscles
extend fully. Breathe the remaining air in your lungs
out of your chest.

2. Turn your head alternately to the right and left,
attempting to look over each shoulder. Holding the
neck between your thumb and fingers, move your
head from side to side again.

3. Let your head droop forwards and nod gently
backwards and forwards then from right to left
several times.

Brow lines

Works on the central part of the frontalis muscle, helping to smooth out horizontal wrinkles of the forehead.

1. Raise your eyebrows, open your eyes wide and stare at a fixed point directly in front of you.

2. Place the tips of your index and middle or ring fingers just above the eyebrows and raise the eyebrows against their resistance.

3. Press three fingers of each hand above the eyebrows lightly and shake the head gently.

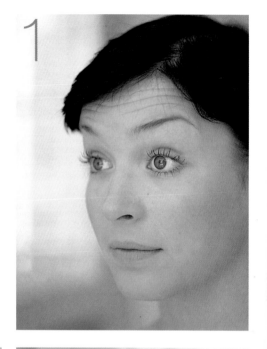

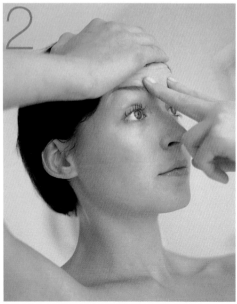

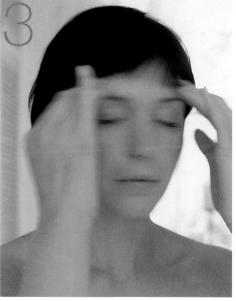

Laughter lines

Works on the quadratic muscles of the upper lip. Helps reduce the prominence of the lines running from the outer edge of the nostrils to the corners of the mouth.

1. Raise the corners of your mouth and upper lip, stretching the top lip up and over the top teeth while opening your mouth about two centimetres. Keep your mouth and neck muscles relaxed. You should feel a tension in the cheek pads.

2. Suck the air into one cheek then move it to the opposite cheek. Then suck air into both cheeks and into the area above your top lip, such that no horizontal or vertical lines are visible. 'Chew' the air. Repeat 5–10 times.

3. Pursing the lips gently, open them about a centimetre as if blowing bubbles and exhale the air gently.

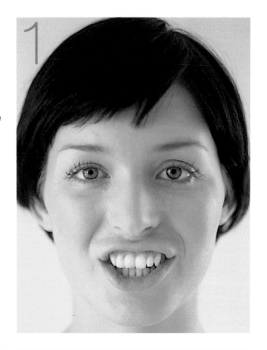

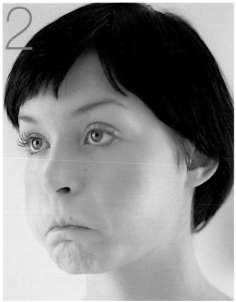

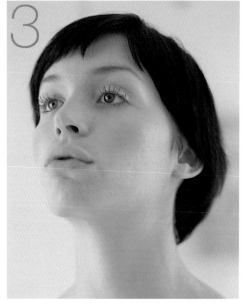

Drooping jowls

Works on the masseter muscle that you use when chewing. Helps to shape the side profile of the cheeks and raise the jowls.

1. Clench your back teeth tightly for 10–20 seconds, increasing the pressure slowly. Feel the muscle contract.

2. Place an index finger on your lower teeth and, holding the finger rigid, pull your teeth up against it. Hold for 10 seconds.

3. Drop your head forward, relaxing the neck, and sway your head gently from side to side as if saying 'no' while looking down.

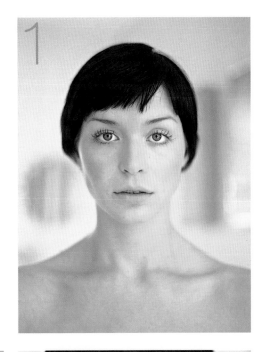

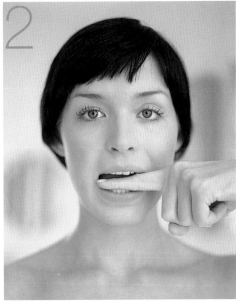

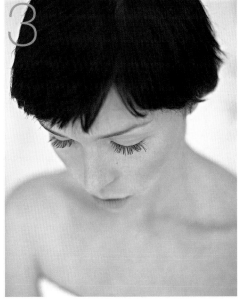

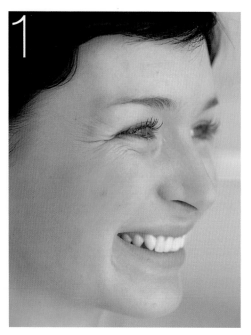

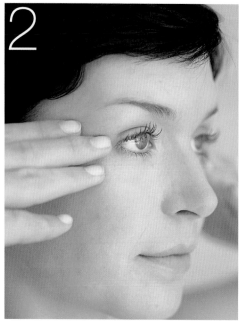

Crow's feet

Works on the outer edge of the eye ring muscle, the orbicularis oculi, which contracts when you laugh or smile causing the characteristic creases.

1. Wrinkle your eyes so that you can clearly see the crows' feet on the outer corners of your eyes.

2. Put your three middle fingers horizontally facing inwards over the skin where the crow's feet emerge.

3. Try to create the crow's feet again against the pressure of the fingertips.

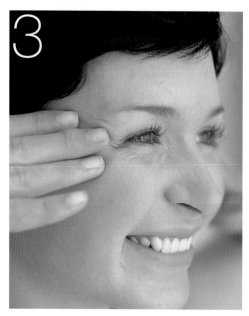

Frown lines

Works on the musculus corrugator gabellae which, true to their name, create the vertical corrugations that form between the eyes when you frown.

1. Frown tightly, then relax the muscles.

2. Put the index, middle and ring fingers of each hand on the temporalis muscle, on the outer edge of each eyebrow, and frown again, feeling the pull on your fingers.

3. Close the eyes and loosely shake out the tension in the muscles by vibrating your fingertips lightly over the muscle.

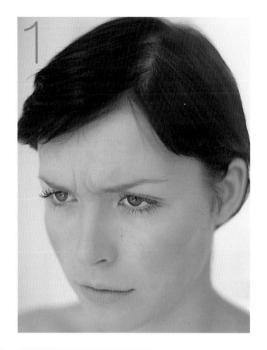

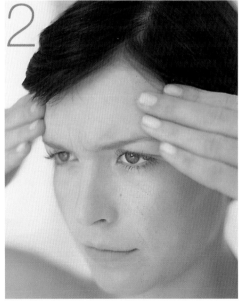

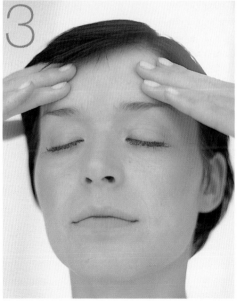

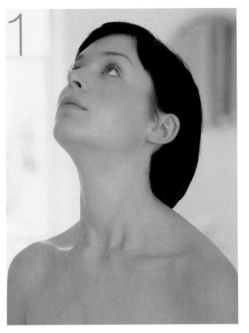

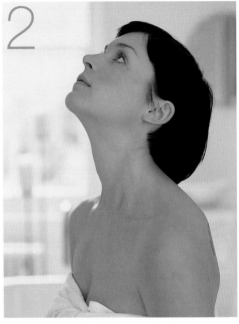

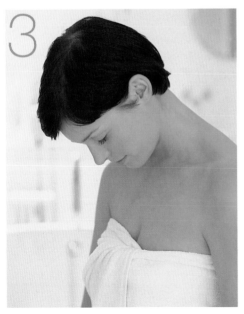

Double chin

Works on the sterno-hyoideus muscle that is connected to the breast bone and which tenses when you chew or stick your chin out.

1. Hold your head upright and tense the shoulder muscles. Roll your tongue back against the roof of the mouth, and press backwards towards your throat, as if swallowing the tongue. If you feel that this movement is over-stretching your skin, open your mouth slightly.

2. Try to swallow. Repeat 4–5 times.

3. Bow your head, open your mouth slightly and slowly move your head from side to side, keeping your jaw loose.

Upper lip wrinkles and sagging cheeks

Works on the orbicularis muscle that runs around the lips and creates creases when you purse them, as well as relaxing the quadratus labii superioris that pulls up the upper lip to form a smile.

1. Push your lips forward into a prominent kiss.

2. Repeat, with your middle fingers pressing against your lips.

3. Blow out your lips like a horse.

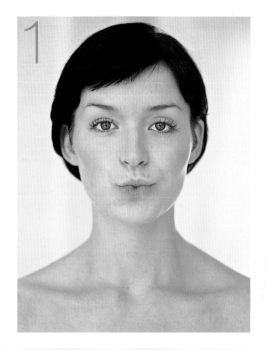

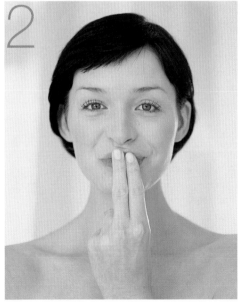

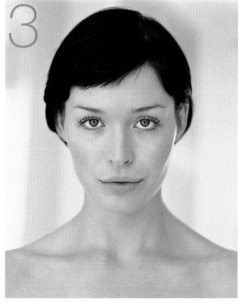

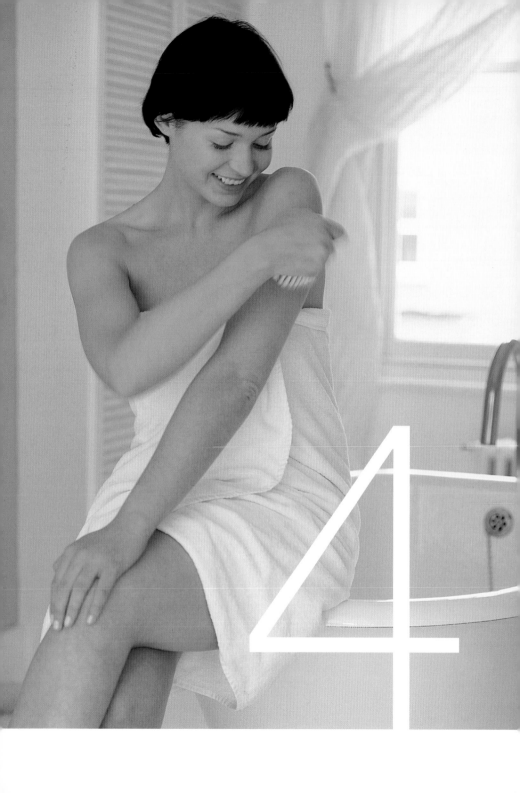

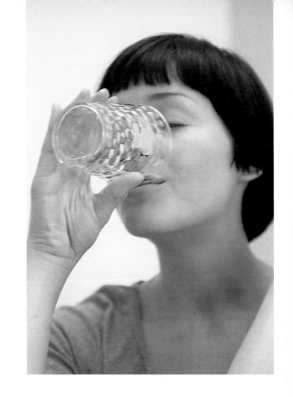

clean up
your act

toxic trouble

Most people think of cleaning their skin as a procedure involving little balls of cotton wool and something runny out of a bottle. It is hardly surprising: manufacturers are continually producing new solutions for skin cleansing, as they prefer to call it. The advent of non-soap bars, foaming washes, pore strips and cleansing gels, to name but a few, have all helped contribute to a huge growth in sales especially among people in their thirties and forties. Cleansers now account for a quarter of all skincare products sold, with sales rising annually.

Cleansers are usually based on mineral oil with added water, alcohol, antibacterials, preservatives, thickeners, fragrances and waxes. Among common active ingredients are allantoins, formulated to soothe but a potential irritant; propyl parabens, included to kill bacteria, but which can cause contact dermatitis; and propylene glycol, included to retain moisture, which often causes sensitivity and on which a ban has been proposed. They do shift grime from the skin, but at a chemical cost.

Outside in versus inside out

More importantly, rather like using a salve to treat a rash, such cleansers are all addressing the issue of skincare from the outside in. Just as an allergic rash is often a symptom of a reaction to a food, skin problems relate to something going wrong inside. Good skin depends on healthy blood getting to the dermis and toxic wastes being filtered away.

If insufficient blood is getting through to the skin, if the blood is carrying a lot of toxins or if accumulated wastes are not getting filtered out quickly enough – in other words, if the system is undernourished or overloaded – it will show in skin problems. They may just be everyday spots, blackheads or rough patches and they may soon disappear with a simple topical treatment. But they are all signs that the skin is stressed and, like other organs, skin ages more quickly under stress.

Organ overload

The skin is the body's largest organ of elimination, filtering out water, urea, ammonia, uric acid and salts through the pores on its surface. It is the liver, kidneys and lymph system, however, which take charge of most waste disposal. But if they are overloaded and unable to complete the job, the skin is used as a dumping ground for the excess, unprocessed toxins.

If the skin is a reflection of the health of the body's circulatory and detoxification systems, it is no surprise that skin problems in general are increasing. An excessively fatty diet, sedentary work, chemically processed food and exposure to airborne pollutants – hallmarks of life in the early 21st century – all gum up the systems that should cart the waste out of the body.

Our bodies have never had it so tough. More than 50,000 industrial chemicals are regularly released into the air and more than 350 million litres of pesticides and herbicides are sprayed on to food and pastures every year.

We obviously do not ingest them all. But if you add up the number breathed in from polluted air, taken as drugs, consumed in water and eaten as pesticides, growth hormones or food additives, it is an alarming toll. And that's not counting the estimated 8–10,000 toxins potentially absorbed through the skin from commercial cosmetic and toiletry products!

Though much feared and discussed these days, toxins are obviously no modern phenomenon. Whether the by-products of natural decay or the results of food digestion, they have always found their way into the body. So it has a sophisticated system for dealing with them (see opposite). But clever though the liver and the lymphatic system are, they are failing to process the sheer number of toxins that most people are confronted with in the 21st century.

Furthermore, our detoxification systems slow down over time – which is why problems caused by toxicity, from deteriorating skin to bowel disorders, tend to increase with age.

Faulty filter

Toxins that fail to get filtered out of the blood cause two major problems for the skin. First, many of them produce free radicals, the destructive oxygen molecules that accelerate the ageing process, leading to the breakdown of connective tissue, thinning of the skin and muscle loss. Second, toxins slow down the circulation of blood, so that they accumulate at a greater rate.

The effects can be particularly apparent in the face. According to oriental medicine, one of the consequences of an inefficient liver is deep furrows between the eyes, while poor kidney function results in puffy bags under the eyes. Spots are another result of toxin accumulation.

So if you have recurrent skin problems, or simply think your skin looks older than you feel, it is worth trying some of the many techniques to increase circulation and detoxify your system.

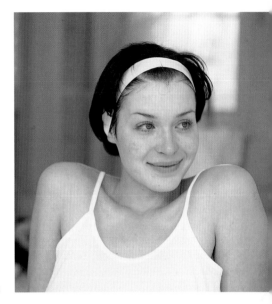

Detox double act

When a harmful substance enters or is produced within the body, the liver and lymph swing into action to neutralize and eject it. The liver deals with substances that the body has metabolized, or burnt up. The metabolism is like a fire, burning up substances and producing harmful smoke. The liver processes this 'smoke', converting its elements into products the body can use, store or eliminate.

This process happens in two stages, which can be seen as getting the rubbish ready for collection and then taking it away. First, enzymes in the liver stick to the toxic molecules and deactivate them. Then the liver produces molecules that transport the waste either into the bloodstream to be filtered out

through the kidneys or mixed with the bile to be released through the intestines.

The lymph glands, meanwhile, produce lymph fluid, which contains white blood corpuscles that absorb dead cells and other waste products. These are carried in the lymph vessels to the lymph nodes, where some wastes are destroyed. The rest are carried to the skin, liver or kidneys to pass out of the body as sweat, faeces or urine.

Skin problems are one of the first signs of sluggish lymph flow. They take different forms, but often manifest themselves in later life in such symptoms as dryness, scaly patches, thread veins and puffy bags under the eyes.

three steps to a spring clean

The detox principle works on two levels. First, the blood and lymph need to be cleared of the toxic sediment they are having to shift around. This means avoiding toxins, giving the gut a break and stimulating the lymph to clear the wastes efficiently. Second, you need to boost your blood circulation. The two processes are reciprocal, with blood and lymph function improving as toxins are cleared and vice-versa. Last of all, if you exfoliate to remove the dead cells and toxins on the surface the results will shine through all the more.

Detoxing

Ideally, detoxing means avoiding ingestion of all pollutants. But short of grafting a filtration mask on to your body, this is impossible today. One way you can get rid of a lot of toxins, however, is combining a detox diet with measures to boost your circulation.

As a form of crisis management, detoxification makes you pay a price. You give up much of what your body depends on yet you do not get a quick fix. As the toxins rise to the surface, your skin may become peppered with blemishes. But cover them up and carry on: within a month at the most they should have made way for new, brighter, smoother skin. It takes around four weeks for the epidermal cells to replace themselves entirely, so be patient.

Boost your circulation

There are many ways of increasing the circulation, some of which can be neatly fitted into your everyday life, others of which take a leap of faith to perform. Start to do four or five from the list over the next few pages regularly and your skin should soon glow with gratitude.

Dry skin brushing Giving your body a firm brush all over has rapid internal as well as external benefits. It stimulates blood and lymph flow, bringing more oxygen and nutrients to the skin surface and carting away wastes via the lymph nodes and skin. It rids the epidermis of dead cells so that the skin can breathe better and encourages new cells to regenerate. It also stimulates the production of sebum, which declines with age. The result is smoother, softer skin.

You need a firm natural bristle brush, such as goat or boar, for the body – preferably one with a long, detachable handle – and a much softer one, or a flannel, for the face.

Starting at your feet and using long, firm strokes, brush the legs then buttocks. Move up to the arms, working from the wrist to the shoulder, and then on to the chest and stomach, brushing more gently where the skin is thinnest. Always brush towards the heart, as it is the area with the largest collection of lymph nodes. The brushing helps to soften any impacted lymph mucus in the nodes and helps to enable it to flow away.

If you work upwards from your feet, your face will be last. Use your soft brush or a dry flannel and soften and shorten your action, as brisk rubbing can stretch or otherwise damage the facial skin.

Brush for 3–5 minutes, every day and preferably before a bath or shower so that the dead cells are washed away. The acceleration of blood flow is quite invigorating, so this is best done in the morning. The difference in your skin should be quite visible after a few sessions.

Epsom salts bath A bath in Epsom salts helps remove toxins at the same time as stimulating the circulation. The magnesium salts draw toxins from the body so they leach out through the skin. You can buy Epsom salts from chemists and some health food stores.

Run a deep, warm (but not hot) bath, tip in a kilo of the salts and agitate the water until they are dissolved. Sit in the bath for 10–15 minutes and massage yourself with a loofah or bath mitt to

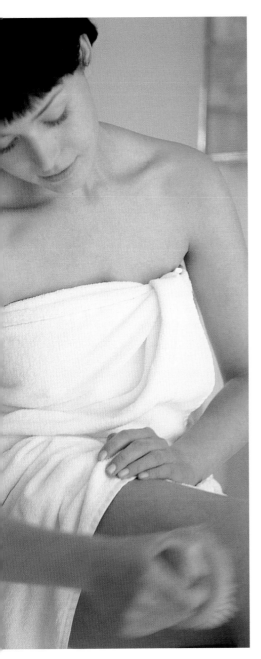

accelerate the effects of soaking. When you get out, dry yourself briskly and wrap up warmly. You will probably sweat a good deal and feel very tired, so preferably have the bath at night. Be sure to moisturize your face, then go to bed with a large glass of water by your side.

Try to do this up to twice a week in your detox period, but not just before or during menstruation as it can increase blood flow.

Essential oils Certain essential oils can help to increase circulation and detoxify your system. They are best applied to the skin during massage, which increases blood flow to the skin manually and helps absorption by creating heat.

The most effective circulatory stimulants are cedarwood, cypress, black pepper, geranium, rosemary and any of the citrus oils. They all have the effect of widening the capillaries under the skin into which they are rubbed. Rosemary is also a lymph stimulant and along with juniperberry stimulates liver function, so if you want to kill two birds with one stone use these in your detox period – but with moderation, since overuse can cause kidney or liver irritation. Both can be safely used on the face if well diluted in a carrier oil or in the bath, when a maximum of four to five drops is needed.

drain the dirt

Lymphatic drainage This is a form of massage which, as its name suggests, stimulates the lymph system into eliminating toxins. It is usually done by a practitioner who will work on key lymph nodes in the neck, armpits, groin, back of the knees and crook of the arms (see pages 122–3).

But almost half our lymph nodes are in the neck area, so it is possible to give yourself a short manual drainage that will have a direct effect on the face.

1. Rub a teaspoonful of oil into the palms of your hands and apply to the neck and face in long sweeping movements. Then using alternate hands, slide up the neck to the jaw bone, covering the whole neck from ear to ear and working lightly over the windpipe.

2. With the index fingers above the lips and middle fingers below, apply a light pressure before sliding the hands outwards to the front of the ears.

3. With the fingers together and hands pointing up the face, apply a firm pressure with the edge of the hand to the area beside the nose and mouth. Release the pressure slightly and, rolling the hands on to the cheeks, slide the hands outwards towards the front of the ears, finishing with a firm pressure.

4. With the index, middle and ring fingers of each hand, start at the inner corners of the eyebrows and slide firmly outwards over the eyebrows.

5. Following on from the last movement, slide the ring fingers lightly inwards underneath the eyes.

6. Close your eyes and with the fingers together, using the whole of both hands, apply a firm pressure to the face holding for a second before releasing. Cover the whole face from nose to ears and from chin to hairline.

7. Cup your hands over your face, closing the eyes, and rest for one minute.

After a manual lymph drainage, the glands in the neck may feel swollen. This is evidence of toxins having moved to the lymph nodes to be drained.

As it is quick and effective, try to give yourself an MLD every day during the detox period.

Herbal help There is a whole range of herbs that help both to stimulate circulation in the blood and to detox the liver. Most can be taken as tinctures or tablets but some can be drunk as a tea or even used in cooking.

The best-established blood boosters are ginkgo biloba, yarrow and rosemary. Using ginger with any of these may enhance the effect as it is believed to increase the bioavailability of the active ingredients in the herbs.

Even humble herbs can be potent cleansers, so it is wise to start off on a fairly low dose, otherwise you could suffer unpleasant reactions as too many toxins are thrown out at once. Take advice from a herbalist or health food shop.

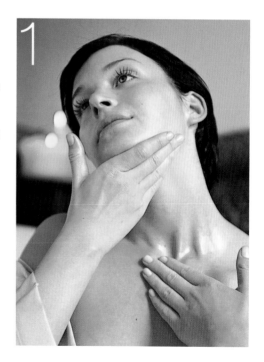

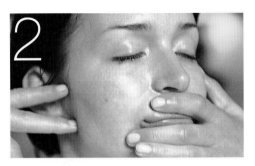

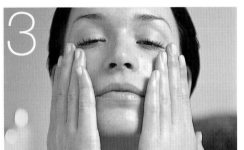

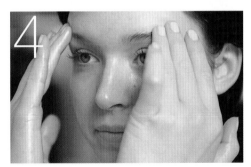

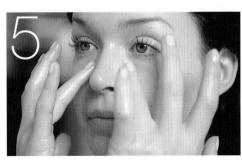

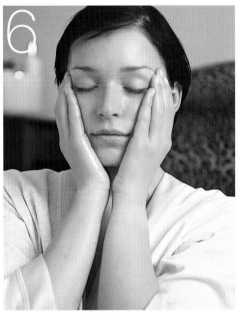

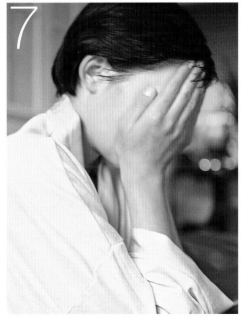

keep it moving

Exercise Minutes after starting to exercise, many of us turn an embarrassingly beetroot tone. That may be bad news for our self-esteem, but it is generally good news for our skin.

Exercise is the single most effective way to boost circulation, as it has immediate as well as long-term effects. In fact, the gradual decline in circulation that occurs with age and is so noticeable in the skin is almost entirely due to a parallel decrease in strenuous activity.

In the first moments of an exercise session, blood supply to the skin actually decreases, as the body feeds the working muscles. But as soon as you start to warm up, it sends more blood to the skin surface, in order to cool the body core down. The whole process is impressively efficient: within a few minutes of starting to exercise, the heart rate triples, blood volume increases sevenfold and the amount of oxygen multiplies by 20, feeding the smallest capillaries in the skin.

Exercise also helps to clean the body out by increasing the elimination of toxins through the lungs in air and through the skin in sweat. Sweating helps not only to clear the skin of debris, but also to lubricate it – a valuable function as it ages and dries.

Exercise greatly benefits lymph flow. Unlike the blood, which has the heart to shift it around the body, the lymph has no internal pump so relies on bodily movement to keep it flowing.

However, do not attempt vigorous exercise at the beginning of a detox diet, as your body needs all its available energy to cope with the dietary changes and restrictions. Gentle stretching, to help toxins to shift, is all that is needed then.

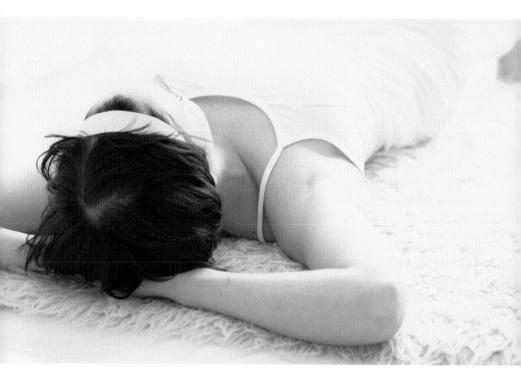

Deep breathing This is something you cannot help doing when you are exercising. But at other times, most of us breathe in a shallow, superficial way that uses only around a third of our lung capacity. Our circulation is compromised and cells do not receive sufficient oxygen to reproduce at their optimum rate – which leads, among other things, to lifeless skin. The image that often springs to mind when we think of deep breathing is of a strident gym teacher exorting children to puff out their chests and pull in their stomachs. Such a posture merely restricts the movement of the abdomen and limits the space in which the lungs can expand, so that they neither take in enough oxygen nor exhale sufficient wastes.

The way to optimize lung function is to relax the stomach and breathe in slowly through the nose, as if you are taking air into the pit of your stomach. This helps relax the diaphragm. Then, in an equally relaxed and measured way, breathe out through the mouth, which enables you to expel toxins more readily. This improves circulation of the blood, enhances lymph flow and massages the liver in a way that stimulates its detox mechanisms. For more breathing exercises, see page 118.

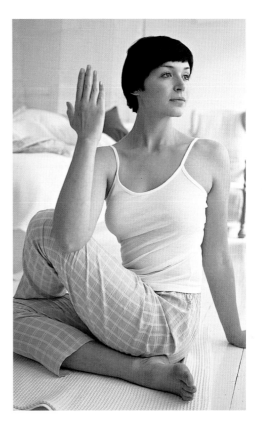

Hydrotherapy This is really a euphemism for cold bathing and not a habit to tell your friends about until the results are sparkling from your skin. They may otherwise believe you to be unhinged!

Although having a cold bath would seem to be more of a spiritual penance than a beauty ritual, it does have a remarkable effect on the circulation. Within three to five minutes of immersing yourself in a cold bath, your blood circulation increases fourfold. Although you may not realize it, your lymph flow is equally boosted.

Apart from widening the arteries, cold bathing also boosts the body's production of white blood cells, destroying circulating toxins, and increases your metabolism so that you burn calories more quickly and feel more energetic.

The water, you may be glad to hear, need not be freezing. In fact, it is best to start at a tolerable 20°C and gradually decrease the temperature over time, as you get used to it (you will!) to 15°C. The bath is the ideal place but you can get a similar effect in the shower. Whichever you choose, try not to hold your breath as that will interfere with your body's adaptation to the cold.

slap happy

Increasing circulation to the face Sometimes, having skipped the cold shower and run out of rosemary oil, you will want a quick-fix circulation solution. Slapping yourself on the face is the best way to get blood into it and is a method routinely used by masseurs. But they call it 'tapotement'. Try the following three-minute routine.

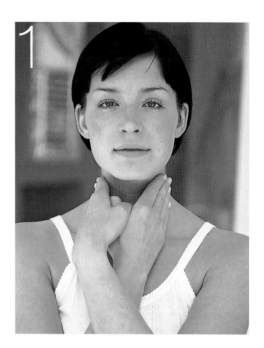

1. Cross your hands in front of the neck and, with the flat of your fingers, tap on the opposite sides of the neck, from the base up to the chin, avoiding the windpipe.

2. Hold the back of your left hand about 4 cm under the chin. With the back of your right hand, tap rapidly upwards on the area under the chin, using the back of the left hand as a 'stop'.

3. With the flat of the fingers and using both hands together, apply firm tapping movements all over the lower part of the face. Start lightly over the mouth and move outwards, covering each cheek and stopping in front of the ears. If you are prone to thread veins, use only light 'piano' movements.

4. Using both hands together and the flats of the fingertips, apply firm tappng movements all over the forehead.

5. Using the hands loosely clenched, 'knock' your head all over with a relaxed movement, varying the firmness of the movement depending on the sensitivity of the area.

6. Using the pads of the fingers, apply deep circular movements all over the scalp from the hairline to the crown, covering the whole head thoroughly.

7. Using your hands alternately, 'comb' through your hair from the hairline to the crown, using long, deep sliding movements.

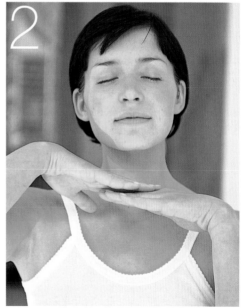

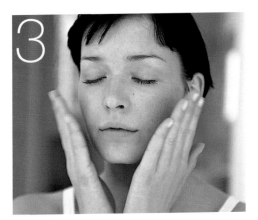

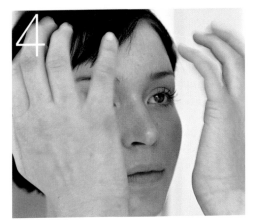

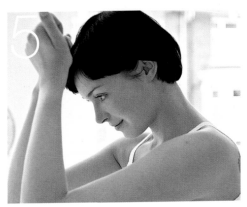

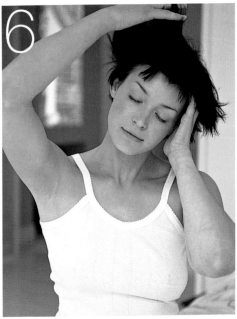

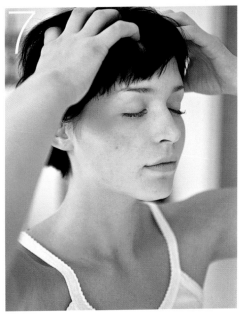

are you intoxicated?

The person who is not carrying environmental toxins in their blood in the late 21st century is living some self-sufficient rural idyll that most of us could only dream of and the rest of us would find numbingly boring. Modern urban life is toxic by definition.

But is your body carrying many more toxins than it is built to handle? There are intrusive and expensive tests to find out, but running through the following questions on your diet and environment will give you a fair idea. You can then decide whether the detox diet (see pages 84–7) is worth it. Simply put a tick or cross beside each.

Diet

Do you regularly consume:
- ☐ Sugary snacks?
- ☐ Tea and coffee?
- ☐ Alcohol?
- ☐ Canned food?
- ☐ Fried food?
- ☐ Smoked or cured meat or fish?
- ☐ Fast food?
- ☐ Tap water?
- ☐ Fluoridated water?
- ☐ Water supplied through lead pipes?
- ☐ Commercially produced (non-organic) fruit, vegetables and meat?

Environment

Do you regularly:
- ☐ Smoke or work with smokers?
- ☐ Take prescription drugs or painkillers?
- ☐ Have amalgam fillings?
- ☐ Use aerosol sprays?
- ☐ Use household cleaners?
- ☐ Exercise near busy roads?
- ☐ Drive in heavy traffic?
- ☐ Work with a VDU screen?
- ☐ Spend a lot of time in the sun?
- ☐ Are you on the pill or hormone replacement therapy?
- ☐ Do you live near electricity pylons or a power station?

If you have more than 15 ticks, you need to reduce your exposure to and consumption of toxins with the detox diet (see page 87). Fewer than ten and you are doing the best you can in the polluted world none of us can escape.

Tips for a healthy liver and lymph

• Avoid any foods to which you suspect you may be allergic. They will produce toxins in the gut that cause stress to the detoxification mechanisms.

• Chew your food well to help release enzymes that aid digestion.

• Toxicity in the body can be caused as much by deficiency of the nutrients the liver needs for detoxification as by exposure to toxins. So make sure you consume plenty of foods containing folic acid, flavonoids, magnesium, iron, sulphate and selenium and B vitamins 2, 3, 6, 12 (see page 95).

• Cut down on stimulants such as tea and coffee, and depressants such as alcohol.

• Eat foods rich in antioxidants, which aid the natural detox mechanisms (see chart on page 95).

• Don't use antibiotics or antacids unless absolutely necessary. Antibiotics can destroy the useful

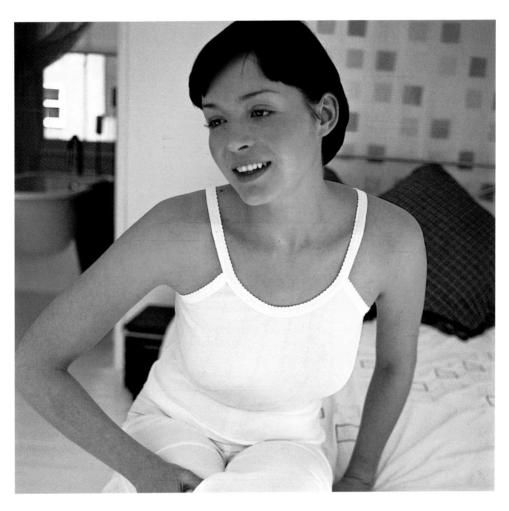

bacteria in the gut that eliminate toxins. Antacids decrease the natural acidity which is necessary for complete digestion.

• Take a daily dose of echinacea, milk thistle or dandelion root, all herbs with a long-established reputation as blood cleansers and skin tonics. They can be taken as tablets, tincture or, if you have an adaptable palate and can learn to tolerate the strong taste, teas.

• Twice a week, take a dose of activated charcoal. This is a medicinal form of charcoal that has the capacity to absorb whatever molecules it encounters, including toxins. But it should not be taken with food or medicines, or it will absorb them.

detox diet

If consuming toxins is inherently a bad thing, then a detoxification diet must by implication be a good thing. But many, if not most, people are truly appalled by the idea. It means not only giving up food and drinks they rely on as social and biological props, but embracing the unfashionable idea of deferred gratification.

The initial shock

The first few days of a detox diet can be an endurance test. You usually feel tired and get withdrawal symptoms from forsaken foods that include muscle pains, mood swings, humdinger headaches and, yes, skin problems. But remind yourself that these are positive signs of the trapped toxins in your body getting released, and persevere: within a relatively short time you will be glowing, even gloating.

Help yourself by choosing the right time. Spring and summer are the ideal seasons to go on a detox diet, as there is a better supply of fresh, locally grown fruit and veg and people feel less need to eat for comfort or warmth. If you work, start the diet on a Friday so you are not wilting over the office desk during the enervating first few days.

Remember, too, you are on a health diet, not a quest for spiritual enlightenment or the ultimate body beautiful. So you only need to follow this regime until the results are reflected back at you in the bathroom mirror.

A diet to suit you

Unlike most detox diets, which set down exact time limits within a strict plan, this one can be adapted to last anything from one to four weeks. The questionnaire on page 82 will help you assess your level of need; the more profound your problem, the longer your diet should be.

So, the plan is split into seven stages. If you are initially trying out just a week-long detox, each stage will last one day, while in a two-week regime each stage will last two days and so on. Obviously, if you choose the longer plan the effects will be greater than if you opt for the one-week version.

Caution This diet is designed for a normal, healthy adult and should not be undertaken without prior consultation with a doctor by anyone who is pregnant, on long-term prescription drugs or has dietary restrictions.

Stage one

Liquids only. Traditionally, this would be just water, which is the quickest and purest means of flushing out the system. It is also thought to stimulate the production of growth hormone from the pituitary gland in the brain, which exerts anti-ageing powers. But adding a squeeze of fresh lemon to warm water helps to stimulate the bowels.

If you find this too restricting even for a day or two, there are other liquids you can take that have supplementary benefits.

Herbal or spice teas can not only ease the tedium of the liquid-only stage but also act as useful detoxifiers or circulatory stimulants. For herbal teas, choose from ginger, dandelion, fennel or yarrow (but alas, you cannot legitimately sweeten them even with health-giving honey).

Juices are another option and if you make them from the fruits that have detox powers (see stage two), all the better. Using a juicer will not only broaden your choices and maximize the nutritional value of the juices, but leave behind a pulp that you can use as an instant face pack (see page 100).

The third option is broth, ideally made from vegetables. However, you can base it on fresh meat or fish stock, which is more important if you have chosen the 28-day diet.

Stage two

Liquid and fruit only. Fruits, though they often taste acidic, are generally very alkaline foods so they help neutralise the acid waste that is produced when you begin to detoxify. With their high fibre content, fruits are also good laxatives and will help shift some of the estimated 3-4 kg of decayed material in the intestines. As with vegetables (stage three), buy organic if you can or you will only be replacing some of the toxins you are eliminating with pesticide residues.

The following fruits all have properties that help during the diet:

Apples contain a lot of pectin, which helps to remove toxins and stimulates the bowel, and tartaric acid, which aids digestion.

Pineapple contains the enzyme bromelin which helps to produce acids that destroy bad bacteria in the gut – encouraging the growth of 'good' bacteria that are important to digestion – and supports the repair of tissues.

Mango contains an enzyme called papain, which helps to break down protein wastes, as well as bromelin (see pineapple, left).

Grapes help to counter the production of mucus, which can clog up tissues, and cleanse the liver and kidneys. Their high fructose content also provides instant energy.

Watermelon is a diuretic, so speeds the passage of fluids carrying toxins through the system.

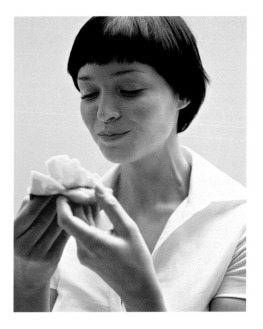

Stage three

Add raw vegetables. Include bean sprouts (best grown yourself), as sprouting increases the nutritional content of seeds fivefold. Use raw garlic, which is an excellent blood cleanser – but at your discretion! Enthusiasts say that if you eat it regularly your breath does not smell, but you need good friends to let you know if that particular theory is borne out in practice.

Vegetables share many of the properties of fruit, and some that can be eaten in salads have particular detox powers:

Fennel helps to improve digestion and also to prevent flatulence.

Watercress contains betacarotene and sulphur, which are both liver tonics.

Dandelion leaves are a liver and kidney tonic and a diuretic.

Parsley is a mild diuretic and contains zinc and trace minerals that aid liver function.

Stage four

Add cooked vegetables and brown rice. Cook the vegetables with as little water and for as short a time as possible to retain their maximum nutrition. Steaming is the best method, followed by stir-frying. Cruciferous vegetables (the ones everyone avoided at school) are particularly good for an overtaxed liver. The rice should always be brown short-grain as it is by far the most absorbent, so soaks up toxins from the gut and is the most easily digested and contains the most fibre.

Include cayenne and ginger among the spices you cook with, as both of these work to stimulate digestion and encourage the elimination of toxins through the skin.

Vegetables normally eaten cooked that have detox properties include:

Leeks, onions and garlic contain sulphur compounds that bind to and speed the elimination of toxic metals.

Globe artichoke stimulates the liver's production of bile, which speeds up digestion.

Jerusalem artichoke contains inulin, which aids the growth of beneficial bacteria in the gut. But beware of their deserved reputation for inducing excessive flatulence!

Beetroot is an acid (as opposed to acid-forming) food that stimulates the production of enzymes in the stomach that aid digestion.

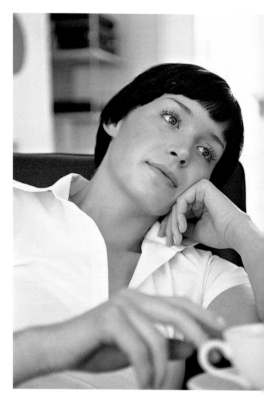

Stage five

Add pulses, nuts and seeds. Pulses are a good source of protein but should not be eaten with rice at this stage as mixing starch and protein can slow digestion. Try to leave four hours between the consumption of the two food types.

Nuts should be eaten raw and unsalted. Like seeds, they provide useful calories in the form of essential fatty acids, which are needed by all the cells in the body but which it cannot manufacture. EFAs also stimulate the flow of bile, which speeds up digestion. Sesame, sunflower and linseeds are all rich sources.

Stage six

Add grains and live yogurt. The yogurt should be goats' or sheeps', which are easier to digest but have the same beneficial action on the gut as live cows' yogurt.

The grains should always be wholegrains, which provide fibre to help move wastes through the intestines and trace minerals useful to liver function. Choose from rye, buckwheat, barley or oats – anything but wheat. All help to deliver a slow and steady supply of glucose into the blood, enabling the liver to build up a supply of glycogen, which it needs to carry out its detox functions effectively as well as to deliver sugar into the blood for an emergency energy supply.

Stage seven

Add fish. Any fresh fish will do but if you choose oily, cold-water fish you will get the benefits for the skin of essential fatty acids. As this is the end of your programme, you should begin to feel more relaxed and not in a hurry to eat everything that you have been missing.

Ideally, introduce your last foods with at least a day between each. By this stage you should be more in tune with your body, which will help you to decide what and when. Add dairy products (cheese, cream, milk) and meat gradually, as they are both high in saturated fats, which slow down digestion. Add wheat last. If you reintroduce these complex foods too quickly, you increase the chances of digestive problems.

Red-light foods (and how to avoid them)

There are certain foods that the human body is poorly designed to deal with. They are those that most often cause digestive or circulatory problems, but unfortunately many are also those on which we are most biologically or socially dependent.

During your detox period, and for a week or two after, avoid all the following, replacing them if necessary with the suggested substitutes:

Cows' milk and its products, such as yogurt and cheese. The fat molecules in cows' milk are too large for many people to digest and lead to lactose intolerance of varying degrees. Try sheeps' or goats' milk equivalents, which have smaller fat moluecles.

Coffee and tea artificially boost circulation, irritate the gut and are acid-forming.

Alcohol interferes with a group of enzymes that are crucial to the detox process, so can act as a 'master toxin' in the body, potentiating the effects of other toxins. It is also a diuretic, so dehydrates skin as well as other tissues.

Wheat often irritates the digestive tract and is mucus-forming. Try bread made from other cereals such as rye and breakfast cereals made from rice.

Lentils often produce embarrassing quantities of intestinal gas.

Mushrooms are a fungus rather than a vegetable and may interfere with the growth of good bacteria in the gut.

Oranges are the most acidic fruit and can congest the liver.

Tomatoes, spinach and rhubarb are high in oxalic acid which can irritate the gut.

Peanuts are a very common allergen and difficult to digest.

scrub and shine

Once you have cleaned up your blood and boosted its circulation, you have probably done more for your skin than any cleansing bar, lotion or gel could. It still needs to be treated topically, as dead cells will continue to accumulate on the surface and grime will still cling to the old cells and natural oils. But if you are expelling fewer toxins and producing healthy new cells more quickly, the process can be very quick, simple – and natural.

Gentle cleansing

You need no more than a flannel, vegetable oil and water. The oil should be one of those that best suits your skin type (see page 35). If undecided, try equal parts of sunflower, avocado and sesame. Run the flannel under the hot tap, squeeze it and press it against your face gently to open the pores. Pour °a little of your oil into the palm of your hand and massage it very gently into your skin, using some of the movements that encourage lymphatic drainage so that you are cleansing on two levels (see pages 76–77).

Having rinsed the flannel, wipe off the oil and accompanying grime thoroughly. Wash the flannel regularly and don't be tempted to use tissues to save labour as they are made from wood pulp and contain microscopic splinters of wood that can get embedded in the skin.

There is a virtue in such simplicity that should show after a week or two of such cleansing. However, every so often, you will need to exfoliate your skin too.

Exfoliation

Exfoliation is not, like cleansing, a daily necessity, but as an occasional treatment brings the benefits of detoxification and better circulation to the surface. It's like the dusting that precedes polishing when you clean furniture: in fact, most household dust is made up of human skin cells. If you do not get rid of those surface deposits first, they will get rubbed around with the polish, producing a smudge rather than a shine. Equally, no cleansing method will make your face glow if there is an accumulation of underlying detritus.

Exfoliation becomes more important with age, as skin cells are renewed more slowly and they have more creases to bury themselves in. Wrinkles packed with dead cells look deeper than those that are cleared out. Moreover, removing these cells speeds up the process of skin regeneration. That is probably why men's skin seems to age more slowly than women's: their daily shave removes not only stubble but dead skin.

Older skin

The older your skin, the gentler a touch it will need. Unlike the rugged stuff on your knees that you can attack with a loofah, the delicate skin on your face is prone to thread veins, irritation or excessive dryness if rubbed too harshly. Some commercial scrubs, as exfoliators are often called, contain rough particles, which although natural can scratch the skin. Others, for example those based on fruit acids, are too aggressive.

The epidermis may be largely made up of dead cells, but it is still metabolically active and if you remove too much of it, it will not serve its protective function of defusing dangerous free radicals from the air or trapping moisture. You can use these harsh new tools when you are young to no apparent ill effect. But they can inflict superficial damage that becomes visible when the skin loses collagen and elastin.

As one skincare manufacturer noted, fine oatmeal or ground almonds are plenty strong enough. Such natural substances from the kitchen cupboard can remove dead cells more moderately and safely than a branded product claiming to do the ultimate scrape-and-shine.

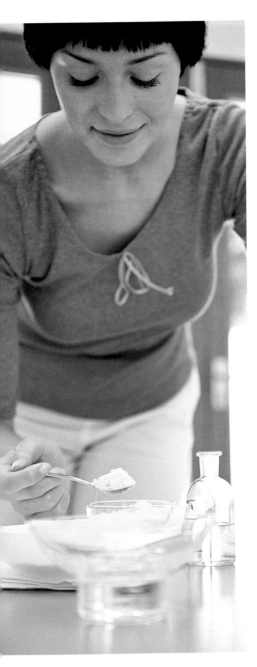

The four most traditional ingredients are salt, which is antibacterial, ground almonds, oatmeal, both traditional cleansers, and sugar, which is now used in glycolic acid preparations. But other granular foodstuffs that are mildly abrasive will do the trick. They do not require special preparation to make them into pastes and can be used just dampened with water for speed. But adding something like cream or yogurt makes them easier to apply, while grape juice will also take dead cells with it when rinsed off.

Experiment with any of the three recipes below to gain the confidence to invent your own.

Oat nut scrub

2 tsp fine oatmeal
2 tsp ground almonds
orange flower water (for oily skin) or cream
    (for dry skin) to blend

Sugar corn scrub

2 tsp cornflower
2 tsp raw brown sugar
1 tsp almond oil
apple juice (for normal skin) or lemon juice
    (for oily skin) to blend

Sticky grape scrub

2 tsp salt
1 dsp grape juice
Greek yogurt to blend

Mix all the ingredients into a smooth paste then leave for five minutes to bind. Gently massage into the face, avoiding the delicate skin under the eyes. Wipe off with a damp muslin cloth, rinse your face in warm water then pat gently dry with a towel.

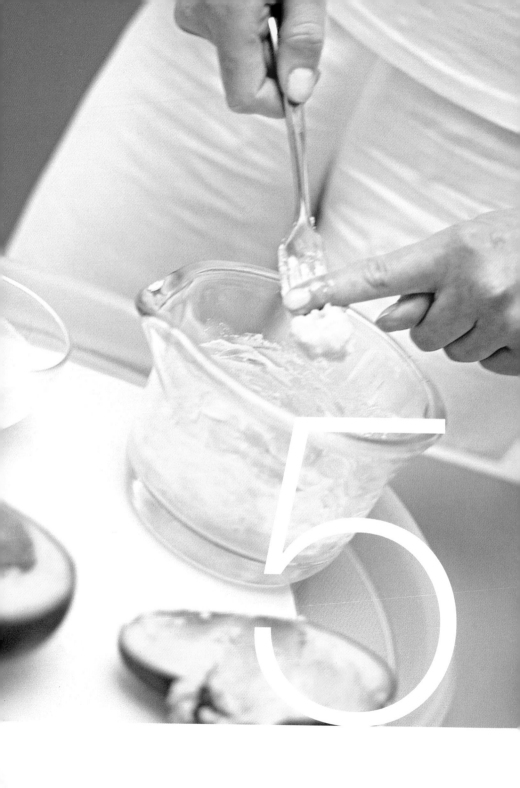

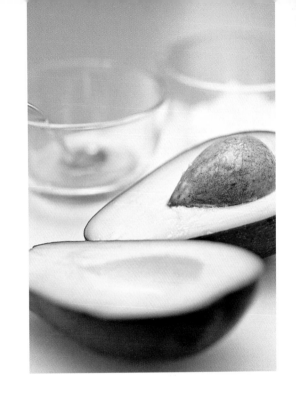

feed
your face

turning inside out

One of the health credos it has been impossible to ignore in recent years is that we are what we eat: our diet influences how we look, how we feel and, ultimately, how we die. Saturated fats contribute to heart disease; alcohol to liver disease; refined carbohydrates to colon cancer... the message has been forcefed to us just like fat pellets are to Christmas geese.

The role of diet

The link between a healthy diet and a glowing skin is rarely acknowledged. Just because it is an external organ, this does not mean that it is not equally affected by what we put inside our bodies. A busy and complex material, like any other in the body, skin needs a precise and complete supply of nutrients to regenerate, repair and defend itself. In effect, what you eat today you wear tomorrow.

Many naturopaths and nutritionists believe that the high prevalence of skin problems today is largely attributable to the fact that, while we are eating more than we used to, many people are eating too many pre-packaged, chemically preserved and calorie-dense foods lacking the essential nutrients that their skin needs.

Manufactured substitutes

It has been left to the skincare manufacturers to raise awareness. With researchers to keep busy and profits to make, they have been only too happy to fill a hole in the market. The result has been a preponderance of creams and lotions containing every vitamin from A to K and phytochemicals to boot. But do these nutrients make it all the way through the dermal layers to where it matters?

The answer is usually no, because they are made up of molecules that cannot penetrate the dense layers of skin tissue. Those that do make it through rely on synthetic chemicals to help them to reach their destination – chemicals that can then be carried into the bloodstream and on to the liver, with uncertain consequences.

Yet manufacturers cannot claim that these substances do penetrate and enter the bloodstream because that would make them transdermal (meaning 'through the skin') and they would have to be classified as drugs. That would mean their being put through comprehensive, long-term, controlled trials to qualify for a medical licence – an inordinately expensive and lengthy procedure.

Meanwhile, health manufacturers have been busy devising vitamin and mineral supplements to do the trick. There is now a whole range of 'oral cosmetics', as they have been called, for skin, hair and nails. (How long before we see tablets claiming to prevent chilblains?)

Eating your way to healthy skin

Though such nutritional creams and capsules may serve some peripheral purpose, it is more effective – and undoubtedly cheaper – to eat what the skin needs from your plate. Eating is the surest way to get nutrients to where they are needed, and if your blood is now detoxified, clean and zipping through even the tiniest dermal capillaries they will get there fast. There are also associated benefits of taking the dietary route, since many of the foods needed for healthy skin tissue are also those that benefit the circulation, digestion and elimination mechanisms.

It is frequently said that you can get everything you need to cure or prevent such-and-such a condition from a 'balanced diet'. But few people really have one these days. As far as the skin is concerned, there are two groups of nutrients that are particularly poorly represented in the modern diet and which are crucial to keeping your skin young. So what is your skin most hungry for?

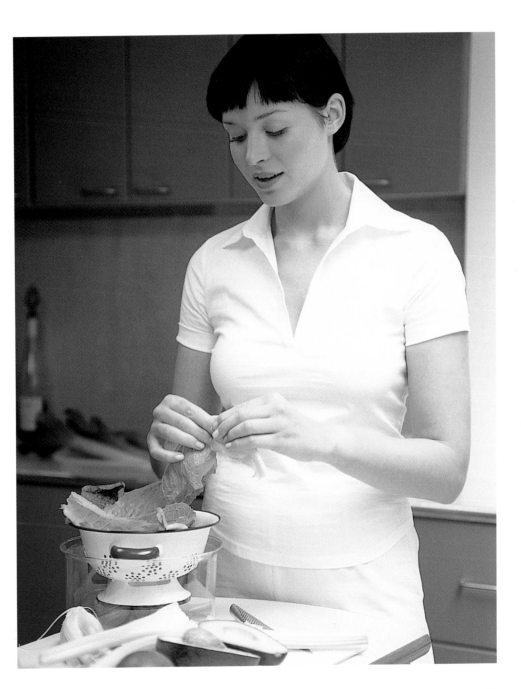

antioxidants

Antioxidants perform such a fundamental role in destroying the free radicals at the root of much age-related deterioration that they can effectively be defined as anti-ageing nutrients.

Free radicals

Free radicals are highly reactive chemicals that get into the bloodstream from polluted air, sunlight and normal metabolic processes. A by-product of oxygen combustion, some free radicals are useful for destroying infection. But many attack cells. They oxidize flesh, scramble molecular make-up and starve the cells of oxygen. In skin, the main victim of free radicals is collagen: its molecules cross-link or fuse together, making it tough and leathery. By the age of 50, it is thought that 30 per cent of cellular protein has been damaged by free radicals. In the skin, the result is wrinkles, bags and creases.

Key antioxidants

Antioxidants slow down the oxidation of tissues by free radicals. More than 100 of them have been identified, but the main ones are betacarotene; vitamins C and E; selenium and zinc. Vitamins C and E and betacarotene are most effective if taken together, as they work in synergy.

Betacarotene is the plant form of vitamin A, which the body converts into vitamin A. It protects against

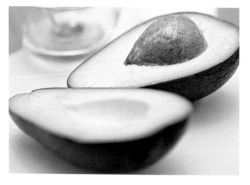

the effects of ultraviolet light, boosts immunity and can protect the skin from bacterial infection.

Vitamin C has a reputation as the most potent antioxidant, and it is recommended for everything from flu prevention to cancer therapy. Vitamin C is also essential for the production of collagen, the elastic tissue in skin that declines with age. Boosting your vitamin C intake will not actually increase your production of collagen, but may slow down its loss.

Vitamin E is probably the best-known skin nutrient. As an antioxidant, it works in tandem with selenium and has the most powerful action against free radical damage caused by the sun. It also helps the skin to retain moisture, to maximize its use of oxygen and to produce new cells where the skin has been damaged.

Selenium protects cells from free radicals and helps to counter dry skin. With vitamin E, it supports the immune sytem, so can help fight infection.

Zinc, like vitamin C, is vital to the manufacture of collagen. It speeds up healing where skin has been damaged, and evens out pigmentation. It is vital to the immune system, so helps to destroy infection. Lack of zinc slows down skin healing and can lead to stretch marks and stubborn blemishes.

Bioflavonoids are a group of 500 compounds or more, some of which are potent antioxidants. They work with vitamin C to protect and condition connective tissue and capillaries.

Proanthocyanidins and anthocyanidins are less well-known members of the antioxidant club. But they can claim élite status. In addition to their own antioxidant activities, they enhance the antioxidant powers of vitamins A, C and E. They are also believed to inhibit the enzymes responsible for the breakdown of elastin and collagen in the connective tissue. A particularly potent form, oligomeric pro-anthocyanidins, are gradually being incorporated into skin creams, but can also be consumed in green tea, turmeric and grape seeds.

Nutrient	What it does	Where to find it	Effect of deficiency on skin
Vitamin A	Antioxidant. Helps to slow down the accumulation of keratin and keep the skin supple	Oily fish; offal; eggs; dairy foods	Scaly skin; flaky saclp; acne; poor wound healing
Betacarotene (pro-vitamin A)	Provides the body with the components to manufacture vitamin A. Protects against the ageing effects of ultraviolet light and boosts immunity	Carrots; dark green vegetables; apricots; oranges; tomatoes; peppers; squash; pumpkin; watercress	As for vitamin A
Bioflavonoids	Antioxidant. Slows down the deterioration of connective tissue and strengthens the small capillaries that feed the skin	Pith and flesh of citrus fruits; apricots; blackberries; apples; cherries; rosehips; buckwheat	Easy bruising; slow wound healing; premature ageing
Vitamin B2	Necessary for the development and repair of healthy skin tissue	Milk; eggs; cereals; mackerel; liver; green leafy vegetables; mushrooms	Seborrhoeic dermatitits or inflammation around the nose and mouth; cracked lips; dull or oily hair
Vitamin B3	Helps the skin produce natural sunscreening substances such as melanin	Brown rice; chicken; wheatgerm; tuna; broccoli	Dermatitis; acne; eczema; fatigue; depression
Vitamin B5 (panthothenic acid)	Necessary for the formation of new skin tissue to maintain healthy hair	Yeast; liver; kidney; eggs; brown rice; wholegrain cereals; lentils	Muscle tremors; cramps; fatigue; anxiety
Vitamin B6	Helps maintain normal oil balance in the skin and prevent allergic reactions	Chicken; yeast extract; beef; broccoli; bananas; wheatgerm	Overactive sebaceous glands, resulting in oily skin; flaky skin; water retention
Vitamin B12	Helps the blood carry oxygen to the skin. Helps eliminate toxins	Red meat; liver; eggs; fish	Dry skin; dermatitis; pale complexion
Biotin	Helps the body use essential fats. Moderates the output of overactive sebaceous glands	Offal; wheatgerm; brewer's yeast	Dry skin; eczema; scaly dermatitis
Vitamin C	Antioxidant. Helps to manufacture collagen. Antibacterial, so helps to reduce infection on the skin. Detoxifies, helping to eliminate waste.	Blackcurrants; strawberries; oranges; cherries; peppers; broccoli; watercress	Broken thread veins; rough, scaly skin; easy bruising; red pimples, dry scalp
Vitamin E (tocopherol)	Helps prevent cell damage. Strengthens blood vessels. Maintains good circulation	Seeds and nuts; oily fish; sunflower oil; avocado; beans; wheatgerm; sweet potatoes	Premature wrinkles; pale skin; acne; easy bruising; slow wound healing
Folic acid	Slows down the loss of moisture from the skin	Brewer's yeast; liver; wheatgerm; molasses	Dry skin; eczema; cracked lips; pale complexion
Calcium	Helps skin regeneration. Maintains good acid-alkaline balance	Milk; cheese; yogurt; parsley; almonds; brewer's yeast	Sallow, 'tired' skin
Magnesium	Works with calcium to build and slow down the age-related shrinkage that produces wrinkles. Essential for muscle activity.	Green vegetables; soybeans; raw wheatgerm; milk; oily fish; wholegrains; seafood; nuts	Constipation, producing sallow and blemished skin; bone shrinkage; lack of energy
Selenium	Antioxidant, so fights free radicals. Helps body use vitamin E. Reduces inflammation	Herring; molasses; tuna; oysters; mushrooms	Dull complexion; dry skin
Silica	Needed for collagen manufacture	Horsetail (herb)	Premature wrinkles; eczema; psoriasis; acne; poor wound healing
Sulphur	Fights bacterial infectin to help keep skin clear. Aids detixificatin by stimulating bile secretion	Lean beef; dried beans; fish; eggs; cabbage	Dull complexion; skin infections; fatigue
Co-enzyme Q10	Supports immune system so fights bacterial infection. Antioxidant, so slows ageing caused by free radicals	Soya oils; sardines; mackerel; peanuts, pork	Depressed immunity; sallow skin
Zinc	Antioxidant. Helps to make the protein that carries vitamin A to the skin. Slows down the age-related weakening of collagen and elastin fibres. Supports the immune system in destroying bacteria	Meat; wholegrains; brewer's yeast; wheatbran; wheatgerm; soy lecithin; beans	Dull complexion; eczema; acne; limp, dull hair; white marks on fingernails

fabulous fats

You can buy any nutrient in supplement form. But your skin will get secondary benefits if you get your antioxidants the old-fashioned way. The foods richest in them are almost all from the greengrocer's.

Watercress, carrots, sweet potatoes and apricots are good sources of fibre, which helps to eliminate toxins by increasing the transit time of food through the gut. Plant foods are alkaline by nature, so help maintain blood circulation by preventing acid crystals in the blood that interrupt flow into the small surface capillaries. Fruit and vegetables are also very low in the fat that slows down circulation and causes spots. That is not to say fat is bad for your skin. It all depends which fats you choose.

Essential fatty acids

After decades of fat phobia, the virtues of these fats is being recognized, which is good news. The most common signs of ageing skin – lack of moisture and suppleness – are also the first symptoms of a deficiency of essential fatty acids (EFAs).

EFAs form part of the fabric of skin cell walls and stem the escape of fluids. They are found in cold-water oily fish, nuts, seeds, wild or organic meats, algae and home-produced eggs. These are the very foods we have eaten less of in the west over the past two or three decades as the proportion of farm-reared animals and processed foods we eat has risen. Ideally, EFAs should account for at least 15 per cent of our calorie intake but in most cases they now account for less than half that.

There are two classes of EFA, known as omega 3s and omega 6s, and it is the former that most affects skin condition and which is most lacking in the western diet. The body cannot make them, so omega 3 EFAs have to come from food. Food manufacturers dislike them because they are unstable, easily oxidized and inclined to go off. If foods containing omega 3s are treated to increase their shelf life, or in the case of oils hydrogenated to

make margarine, their beneficial properties are lost.

A quick way of increasing your dietary intake of EFAs is to use sesame, rapeseed, walnut, soybean or flax oils in the kitchen. They are very rich in EFAs and are prone to go rancid, so must be kept in the fridge. They are also an acquired taste. A palatable alternative is eating tinned oily fish, which will also slow down the loss of minerals from your bones, a process which begins in one's thirties and which by one's fifties is visible in the face as skin wrinkles around the shrunken bone. At the same time, decreasing your intake of saturated and processed fats also helps as these compete with and cancel out EFAs in the body.

Reasons to up your intake of EFAs

It takes four to eight weeks for the effect of EFAs to show in the skin, but it is a big difference. Your skin will feel less tight after washing or exposure to the elements and its surface will be softer and dewier. In the longer term, a diet high in EFAs will defer, if not prevent, the appearance of wrinkles.

Increasing your intake of EFAs has secondary benefits. They help to improve circulation by increasing the flexibility of blood cells, enabling them to get into the capillaries that carry oxygen and nutrients to the skin; and decrease food cravings.

Don't worry about the extra calories in oily fish, nuts and seeds – EFAs speed up your metabolism, helping you to burn calories more quickly – so are associated with a decline rather than an increase in body fat. Neither will upping your EFA count make your skin greasier, since their molecules disperse rather than stick together like those in saturated fats, so do not clog the pores in the same way.

Supplementary benefits

The enthusiasm for food supplements prevalent in the past two decades remains unabated. No sooner has a food scientist revealed the virtues of a nutrient than a supplement manufacturer quickly concentrates it into a capsule or tablet.

This is pill-popping of the best kind, but is it really necessary? Most nutrients are readily available from foods. The following few, which are widely deficient in our diet, should be the only supplements you need to consider taking for skin health.

Vitamin E The typical western diet is not rich in vitamin E, which is destroyed by chlorinated water, airborne pollutants, and oestrogen. So it may make sense to take a supplement. But make sure it contains natural vitamin E (d-alpha-tocopherol), which is more effective than the synthetic version (dl-alpha-tocopherol).

Essential fatty acids If you cannot eat enough seeds, are allergic to nuts and don't like the taste of EFA-rich oils, take a supplement of evening primrose oil or borage oil, which are widely available.

Co-enzyme Q10 Deficiency of this antioxidant, which helps skin repair and boosts immunity, is not uncommon because it is easily destroyed by caffeinated and alcoholic drinks and sugar.

Selenium Many Europeans are short of selenium because the wheat in Europe contains little. Offal is a good source, but we eat less of it. On average we get only half the 60–70 mcg a day recommended.

Glutathione This is a powerful detoxifier and antioxidant synthesized in the body from three amino acids. All these are found in fruit and vegetables, but they are most effective if taken together, which is easiest in supplement form.

Silica The body's ability to store this nutrient declines with age. Unless you can take the taste of horsetail tea, a supplement is a good idea.

Too much of a good thing?

All these nutrients, and those listed in the chart (page 95) benefit the skin in some way. But once your body has enough vitamin C to make collagen, enough A to make keratin or enough E to pitch

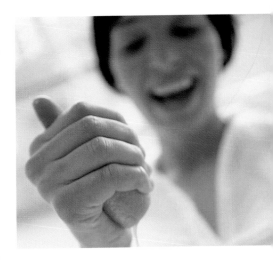

battle against free radicals, there is no benefit in taking more. In fact, an excess of some non-water-soluble nutrients can produce skin problems of a different kind. So don't be taken in by claims that nutrient x, y or z will radically rejuvenate your skin: it is a human organ and has its limits.

Foods to limit or avoid

Saturated fats make the blood cells less flexible, reducing their ability to squeeze into the tiny capillaries that feed the skin. They also increase the risk of clogged pores in people with oily skin.

Sugar increases the frequency and severity of bacterial infection on the skin, as the bacteria feed off the sugar.

Fried, smoked or barbecued food. These cooking methods all destroy antioxidants in food.

Salt draws water out of body cells, drying tissues including the skin.

Tea, coffee and alcohol encourage the elimination of water through the kidneys, drying out skin tissue.

Alcohol interferes with liver function, so facilitates the build-up of toxins, which are often pushed through the skin.

kitchen cosmetics

Facial feeds are designed to bring about a quick improvement in the condition of your skin. They have been used since antiquity as a facial first aid that, if repeated regularly, also has cumulative benefits. Many of the basic ingredients that are used in commercial packs are derivatives of everyday materials people once grew or dug up to convert into skin feeds. The formulae may have changed, but they still work according to the same ancient principles.

Basically, if you apply something to your skin that dries at room temperature, it will tighten the skin. If you include an acidic substance, it will exfoliate and tone. If the main ingredient is rich in natural oils, it will nourish and lubricate.

Home-made face packs can visibly improve your complexion by increasing local blood circulation, neutralizing bacteria, stimulating the elimination of wastes, trapping moisture on the surface, or firm up by closing the pores. The ingredients are readily available, inexpensive and are unlikely to cause allergic skin reactions.

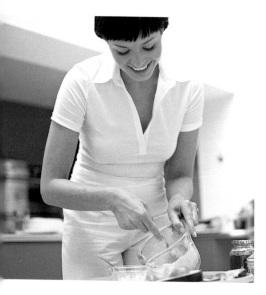

Basic ingredients

Clay has been a staple of face packs for centuries. A mud it may be but it is also a ruthless cleanser that can draw impurities rapidly out of the skin. It also absorbs excess oil and tightens the pores, leaving the skin silky and even-textured. As an anti-inflammatory, it does not cause allergic reactions.

Fuller's earth is probably the most widely used clay in face packs and, despite its grim colour, has strong cleansing properties. White kaolin has a strong astringent effect, so firms up the skin while boosting blood and lymph flow.

But it is probably green clay that is of most interest to people trying to hold back the ravages of time, since its repeated application seems to stem the spread of wrinkles, probably by stimulating the surface muscles of the face along with lymph and blood flow. Green clay seems both to normalize oily skin and enrich dry skin.

If time is precious, clay mixed with water (floral or spring) and a few drops of essential oils forms the basis of the quickest and simplest face mask.

Flour is used to bind ingredients. But, chosen carefully, it can also nourish and cleanse. Gram flour is used as a cosmetic staple all over the Indian subcontinent. But other flours, such as corn, oat or wheat, can be used.

Kelp has similar effects to clay and can refine the skin by tightening the pores. It is a very rich source of vitamins and minerals. But it does have a uniquely fishy smell, so requires essential oil to give it the aroma of a cosmetic rather than something dragged off the harbour.

Brewer's yeast has extractive properties, so can cleanse and help oily skin in particular. It is also a good binding agent.

Turmeric is an Asian staple and traditionally used in pre-nuptial face masks for that special glow. An antiseptic, it can clear the complexion as well as soften the skin.

Yogurt Live yogurt will, true to its name, liven up your skin. It contains lactic acid which helps to draw oil and bacteria out of the skin while drawing moisture in. It also tones and tightens the skin. Used regularly, it may help to prevent spots by balancing the skin's acidity.

Honey hydrates the skin. It is found in many moisturizing face packs for dry skin. Its mildly antiseptic properties also mean it can help oily skin.

Pollen grains are rich in amino acids, vitamins and minerals. They used to revitalize ageing skin, any effect of the nutrients being enhanced by the exfoliating effect of the grains.

Egg is a double blessing. The white is good for closing pores and firming the skin, while the yolk, which contains a lot of fatty acids, lubricates and nourishes. They are usually used separately.

Aloe vera is a plant which has been used for its healing properties for thousands of years. The liquid or gel which is extracted contains active enzymes reputed to diminish wrinkles.

Vegetable or nut oil are both used as emulsifiers which can moisturize, nourish and smooth.

Flower water is a mixture of distilled water with essential oils added. The most popular in skincare is rosewater; its slight acidity makes it a good toner. Orange flower water is used to balance oily skin.

Floral water (also called hydrolats) is the liquid left when essential oils are distilled and is used to tone and rebalance. It is used in masks or dabbed on to the skin after removing one. Fennel is traditionally used to prevent or combat wrinkles; marigold has a reputation as a good moisturizer for ageing skin.

Fruit and vegetables

Plant foods are rich in a variety of enzymes believed to stimulate the skin cells. Whether or not they can penetrate enough to make long-term difference is open to debate, but they can certainly leave the skin tingling and glowing. Fruit, albeit in a highly condensed and synthesized form, is a key ingredient in the glycolic acid 'face peels' that have become so popular. Home-made face packs contain much more of the goodness from the fruit than processed shop-bought ones.

For dry or mature skin

Avocado is rich in the monounsaturated oils easily absorbed by the skin and in vitamin E. **Grape** has the trace elements believed to stimulate new skin cell growth and its acid juice helps exfoliate. **Carrot** is rich in betacarotene and a good moisturizer, but it is watery, so needs a binding agent. **Papaya** contains papain, a plant enzyme that helps dissolve dead skin. **Blackcurrant** helps hydrate dry skin.

For normal skin

Peach is soothing and a mild lubricant. **Pineapple** contains bromelin, an enzyme that helps break down protein wastes in the gut and is thought to dissolve wastes on the skin. **Tomato** is very alkaline so helps to moderate skin acidity while acting as a mild emollient. **Banana** is rich in starch and sugar and a good solid basis for a calming and nourishing mask. **Apple** contains pectin, which is a powerful detoxifier and mild antibacterial, so benefits oily skin.

For oily skin

Pear helps to encourage the elimination of wastes through the epidermis. **Lemon** launches a two-pronged attack on oily skin. As an astringent antiseptic it helps to neutralize bacteria and close pores, while the vitamin C in it accelerates healing of spots and blemishes. **Cucumber** contains the ascorbic acid esterase which acts as an astringent to close open pores. **Apricot** contains vitamin PP, which is a strong bactericide and astringent. **Strawberries** contain salicylic acid, which is used in commercial fruit acid peels, and is an astringent so helps to balance oily skin.

making up a facial feed

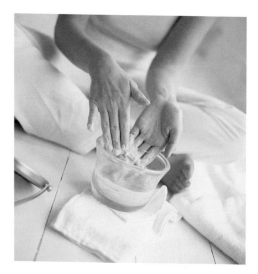

The most important thing is get the consistency right: too sloppy and you will be lying down to keep it in place; too firm and you risk damaging the skin as you scrape off the crust.

To produce a mask, you normally need some fluid, a binder and oil. The fluid may be ready-supplied in the fruit or vegetable you use; if not, you can add floral or plain water. If the latter, spring or distilled water is best; if you use tap water, filter and preferably boil it first to remove the hard deposits and impurities.

If your chosen base is fruit or vegetables you will need a blender or liquidizer to reduce the flesh to a fine pulp; otherwise you risk turning your face into a temporary compost heap. You can then use the blender to incorporate the remaining ingredients. Always wash or peel fruit and vegetables. If using plant foods or yogurt, or both, you may need some powdered clay or flour to bind it together.

When including oil, add it last and drip it in slowly so that it has a chance to emulsify, much as you would if making mayonnaise. Adding a capsule of evening primrose or borage oil will give the mixture

an anti-ageing edge as they help to kill free radicals and to retain moisture.

The oil most commonly used in traditional face masks is almond, but almost any will do. Choose yours according to your skin type (see page 35).

Applying the feed

First make sure your skin is squeaky-clean and if necessary exfoliate (see page 88). Otherwise, the surface residues or dead skin cells will interfere with good absorption. To enhance the effects of a facial feed, massage it into the face methodically, using some of the upward and outward movements from the routines on pages 36–45. It needs to be left on for a minimum of ten minutes. If it has not done its job after 20, it never will. Then rinse it off with warm water, using a clean flannel or muslin cloth if the mixture has solidified.

If you want the full treatment, then apply a toner afterwards. A flower water such as rose or orange is ideal and you can enhance its effect by adding an appropriate essential oil. Bergamot, cypress or juniper are all good for toners, but you could use any from the list on page 35 for your skin type.

Then leave it at that, and don't be tempted to put on make-up to complete the picture. If allowed, skin uses two to three per cent of the body's total oxygen by direct absorption from the air and gets rid of at least as much carbon dioxide waste the same way. Both revitalize it. So just as you rest after a meal, after a good facial feed give the skin a respite and let it respire.

The four recipes below are just examples of some of the facial feeds you can make at home.

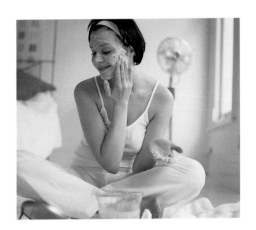

Turmeric and egg feed

The essential fats in the egg yolk and softening properties of turmeric make this a luxurious facial feed for tired and dry-to-normal skin.

1 egg, separated   *2 tsp turmeric*
2 tsp brewer's yeast   *2 tsp pollen grains*
2 dsp jojoba oil   *rosewater to blend*

Whisk the egg yolk and then add the remaining ingredients. This feed is easy to apply but rather sticky, so sponge off carefully and it will leave your skin beautifully smooth.

Egg firming mask

Combining the tightening properties of egg white, the refining qualities of kelp and the astringent, firming action of geranium oil can take years off your face – for an evening, anyway.

1 egg white   *4–6 tsp kelp*
1 drop essential oil of geranium

Lightly whip the egg white until it is white and bubbly but not stiff. Thoroughly mix in the kelp powder and essential oil. Smooth thinly over the face and wait for it to dry thoroughly before wiping, then rinsing it off.

Refreshing toner

After applying some facial feeds, your skin may feel in need of light refreshment. A simple, but very effective and refreshing toner can be made from a flower water, such as rosewater, combined with small amounts of an appropriate essential oil or two. The recipe below is for dry-to-normal skin. For normal-to-oily skin, replace the rosewater with orange flower water and the essential oils with bergamot and cypress.

100 ml (3½ fl oz) rosewater   *1 drop lavender*
1 drop frankincense

Mix the liquids thoroughly by shaking them in a small jar. Saturate a piece of cotton wool and dab lightly all over the face.

Avocado and honey nourishing mask

The rich oils in avocado, humectant quality of honey and stimulating effects of the essential oils make this a good feed for dry, ageing skin.

quarter of a ripe avocado
1 tsp runny honey
2 tsp live Greek yogurt
2 drops jasmine or rose otto

Mash the avocado very thoroughly with a fork, then stir in the remaining ingredients. Apply quite thickly to the face and leave on for at least ten minutes. Wipe off with a dry muslin cloth, then rinse the cloth in warm water to remove the rest of the mask. After such a rich mask, it is a good idea to perk up your skin with a refreshing toner, such as the rosewater mix below.

Cucumber and clay tonic

The astringent properties of cucumber and clay make this a good tonic for normal-to-oily skin.

5 cm (2 in) piece of cucumber
4 tsp green clay   *2 tsp brewer's yeast*

Put all the ingredients in a blender and mix until smooth. If a little watery, add another teaspoon or two of clay.

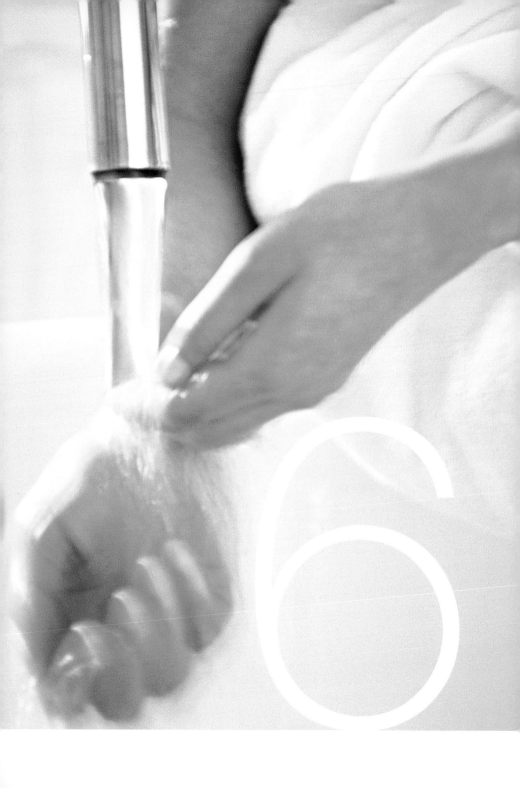

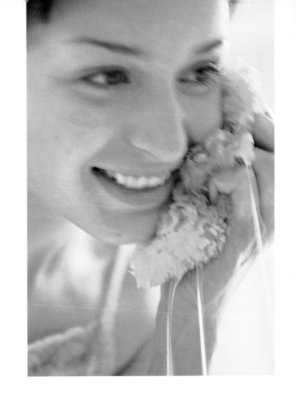

is your
skin thirsty?

liquid assets

The face attracts more poetic and lyrical descriptions than any other part of the body, bar perhaps the heart. If attractive, it is frequently compared to a flower or fruit: a peaches-and-cream complexion; the look of an English rose; the blooming skin of a pregnant woman. 'Beauty is but a flower which wrinkles will devour,' warned the poet Thomas Nashe (1567–1601): some things don't change over four centuries. Like a plant, the skin on the face needs one thing more than any other to flourish: water.

Dehydration

In a certain sense, the face is no different from any other part of the body, which is composed of two-thirds water. Dehydration in other organs of the body can cause a whole spectrum of problems, but the consequences are all invisible. By contrast, dehydrated skin manifests itself to the world in wrinkles, bags and bulges.

Just as a balloon needs air to keep its membrane taut and bouncy and its shape regular, so the skin needs water to fill it out. Deprive either of the material that keeps them buoyant and they collapse downward and inward.

Skincare manufacturers like to convince us that there are at least six different skin types (a list that seems to lengthen as time and commercial ingenuity progress). The traditional preparations for dry, normal or oily skin are now joined by those for 'sensitive', 'combination', 'mature' and the catch-all 'problem' skin. But, while many of us might feel we fit into those neat diagnoses at times, as the years roll by we nearly all develop one and the same skin type: dehydrated.

Throughout history women have tried all manner of unpleasant treatments to rehydrate their skin. The Elizabethans drenched their faces in bean water, rain water and urine, while 17th-century beauties sacrificed small birds to make 'Pigeon's water'.

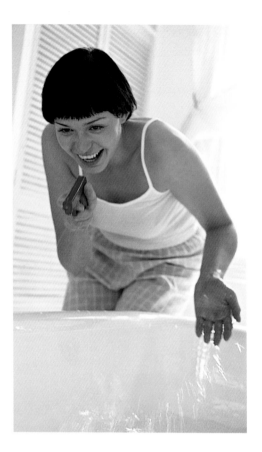

Great escape

Sadly, dehydration is (yet another) part of the natural ageing process. With age, the skin thins, with the effect that more moisture can evaporate through it. Already bearing the thinnest skin on the body, the face loses proportionately more moisture than its depth dictates because it is also the most exposed part of the body. The thinning process goes on imperceptibly from one's thirties but accelerates at the menopause. One reason that men's skin tends to age more slowly is that it is thicker to start with so retains more moisture and does not suffer this hormonal insult.

With age, you also perspire less and produce less sebum. While sweat and oil do not sound like a recipe for beauty, they are great guardians of moisture. Facial oil produced by the sebaceous glands does not lubricate the skin like teak oil on an old table top. Like sweat, it prevents water escaping from it by providing a surface seal. Yet even a twenty-something aerobics addict with oily skin will find that time dries out her face more quickly than her ankles, buttocks or belly. While the shape and texture of the deflating balloon happens noticeably in a few days, the dehydration of the skin happens so slowly it is imperceptible, except with hindsight.

Panic purchase

Most women respond to the ongoing crisis, somewhere in their thirties or forties, by stocking up on more moisturizers. Demand for them has risen 50 per cent in the past five years, which is a likely reflection of the ageing population as well as higher-tech creams sold on the back of often pseudo-scientific claims.

They prove a persuasive pitch to the ageing consumer with money to spend: moisturisers now account for more than half of all skincare products sold, reaching a peak in the 40–50 age bracket.

British consumers spend nearly £400 million a year on moisturisers in an effort to refresh their thirsty skin. Yet, despite their name, they do not primarily put moisture into the skin. The epidermis can absorb relatively little and its capacity for absorption declines with age, as its proportion of keratin increases. Rather, moisturizers are a sort of sebum-and-sweat substitute designed to stop water escaping.

Traditionally, there are two kinds: oil-in-water and water-in-oil emulsions. In the first, the microdroplets of oil are held within the water, resulting in a light and runny cream; in the latter, the water is held in the oil, which gives the cream a richer consistency.

The runnier moisturizers may feel as if they are hydrating the skin more, but the effect is very temporary since most of the water applied to the skin surface will evaporate. You can get a similar effect by splashing or spraying your face with water.

Furthermore, even what oil-in-water creams achieve comes at a cost. Because they contain a lot of water they require more preservatives to prevent bacteria multiplying. The most common is hydroxy-benzoic acid, which in the short term can cause irritation and in the long term can build up in the body with unknown effects. A ban has been proposed on it in the US.

But skincare manufacturers only too ready to cash in on an expanding market are producing alluring new preparations sold on the back of ever more inventive technological claims. So conventional oil-and-water creams have been joined by those containing liposomes, nanospheres and other systems designed to carry water into the skin.

However sophisticated the technology behind the creams, all efforts are focused on the external symptom rather than the internal cause. Yet it is deep within the dermis, whose cells are 80 per cent liquid, that water is needed. Each molecule of protein in the gel-like ground substance that supports the skin's connective tissue is designed to absorb 1,000 times its weight in water.

As with food, so with water: the greatest benefits come from consuming it rather than attempting to apply it, by whatever means, to your face.

use it or lose it

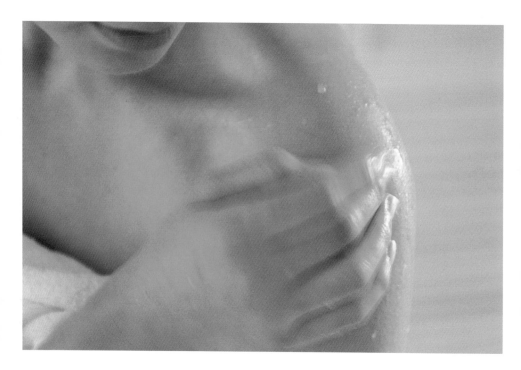

In the course of a normal day, without breaking sweat, the average body loses at least 1.5 litres of water through the skin, lungs, gut and kidneys. It has to do this to eliminate toxins – among them those that cause dark bags under the eyes and those that congregate under the skin to erupt as spots. At the same time as it is expelling water, the body also needs to produce a third of a litre of water to burn glucose for energy.

The amount of water we use and lose obviously varies from one person to another, according to their size and level of activity (see opposite). But it follows that the average person needs to take in at least two litres of water a day to function optimally.

Few people drink anything like that quantity. It may seem as if you do. But social custom dictates that a lot of liquid is drunk as coffee, tea, beer, coke and saccharine-sweetened sodas. All are diuretics,

so much of the liquid you take in enters the sewerage system within an hour or two of putting down your cup. It does not have time to hydrate brain cells, let alone be absorbed by the dermis, which comes very low down the list in the body's order of priorities.

Consequently, most people, without knowing it, are chronically dehydrated. The effects, while hardly life-threatening, can greatly impinge on everyday activity. Fatigue, headaches, indigestion and joint pain are the most common symptoms of dehydration, though we usually attribute them to other causes.

Thirst first

But if your body is so short of liquid that its protests hurt, how come you don't feel permanently thirsty? Simple: when you deprive the body of water, it blunts the thirst mechanism. The message to the brain to drink is interrupted, probably as a survival measure to adapt in the short term to drought. But in the longer term, the brain accepts moderate water shortage as the norm.

Children are different. Water constitutes a greater part of their body tissue and they tend to breathe out more of it. So they have a sharp and sensitive thirst mechanism to match, which is why they drink a lot and guzzle, rather than sip, drinks. The mechanism naturally declines from one's late teens or early twenties, but what blunts the sensation of thirst most is simply not drinking enough.

Recognizing thirst

Once you start drinking more, you will notice that the natural mechanisms are re-awakened and you begin to thirst for more. Within a short time, you want the amount of water your body really needs. But oddly, you may never feel a dry throat, as that is one of the last symptoms of dehydration, not the first.

When the body needs water, it sends out messages through various systems which manifest themselves as subtle symptoms. It may be a tingling in the nasal tract or an incipient sense of fatigue. The symptoms of thirst are quite individual, and you begin to recognize them as you follow your instincts. It is not difficult once you start, since the benefits – including an increase in energy – are so tangible. And fear not: following those instincts will not have you rushing to the toilet constantly, since your bladder capacity will increase as you drink more.

The added benefit

The benefits for the face of drinking more are not just an increase in water supply to the dermal cells to plump them out. There are many secondary effects. A further aesthetic consequence is that drinking more water often makes you lose weight.

This is an unexpected, but often welcome, side-effect that results from getting in touch with your thirst mechanisms. When energy levels are low in the body, the central control system in the brain registers the sensations of hunger and thirst simultaneously. Programmed from infancy to associate sweet tastes with energy, most of us reach for, at best, a banana and, at worst, a biscuit. Only by drinking water rather than snacking when you feel a need for energy will your body learn the surprisingly subtle difference between the sensations of hunger and thirst.

How thirsty is your body?

You can work out how much water your body needs on an average day by doing a very simple calculation. Divide your weight in kilos by eight, then round up the figure. For example, if you weigh 60 kilos the answer is seven-and-a-half, so the end figure would be eight. That is how many glasses you need a day – equivalent to around two litres.

An alternative guide, using imperial measures, is to halve your body weight in pounds. That is how many fluid ounces you need in a day. So if you weigh nine-and-a-half stone or 132 lb (equivalent to 60 kilos) then you end up with 66 fl oz. Divide that by eight (the number of fluid ounces in an average glass) and round the figure down. Again, that gives you eight glasses or four pints.

Both of these 'answers' are the minimum number of glasses you need on a day of normal activity in cool weather. When the sun is out and you are digging the garden or jogging, you will need to add half as much again.

Don't forget that you can eat water too. Some fruitarians, who live on a pure fruit diet, drink nothing from a cup or glass. Most fruit and vegetables consist of about 90 per cent water, and four pieces of fruit and four servings of vegetables (just over a kilo in weight) can provide a litre of water.

water works

Rehydrating your body by drinking more water can enhance your skin in more ways than one:

• In people with dry-to-normal skin, it stimulates the sebaceous glands into producing more oil, which traps in more moisture. But don't worry: it will not make oily skin more oily.

• The kidneys are flushed out more effectively, so fewer toxins travel to the skin's surface.

• The muscles, in the face and elsewhere, become more powerful and flexible. They should be three-quarters water and if they lose just three per cent of that they lose ten per cent in strength.

• The connective tissue becomes less rigid as it is hydrated so the gelatin in which it is grounded becomes more flexible and facial expressions become less fixed.

Bottled or tap?

Fears about the quality of the water that repeatedly negotiates the sewerage network before spurting out of our domestic taps have fuelled a boom in

sales of the bottled variety. In the past decade, sales of mineral water in the UK have almost tripled.

In principle, there is good reason to swap tap water for bottled. Hundreds of chemical contaminants have been identified in tap water, the most common being nitrates, lead, aluminium and pesticides. But bottled water is not always the pure and simple substance it sounds.

Bottled water can be classified as table water, spring water or natural mineral water. Only the last is guaranteed to be from an unpolluted underground source and is untreated. 'Spring water' is usually subterranean too but it does not have to be bottled on the spot and might well be treated to remove bacteria. 'Table water' is the least well-defined and could be a mixture of water from many sources, including tap water. However, it has usually been purified and often has minerals added.

But don't think of mineral water as a liquid nutritional supplement. Spring or tap water is often artificially carbonated, a process that can cause

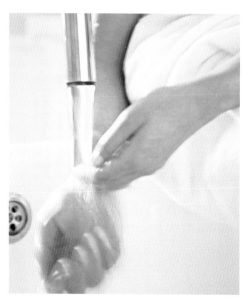

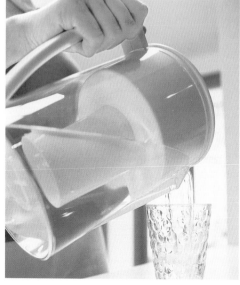

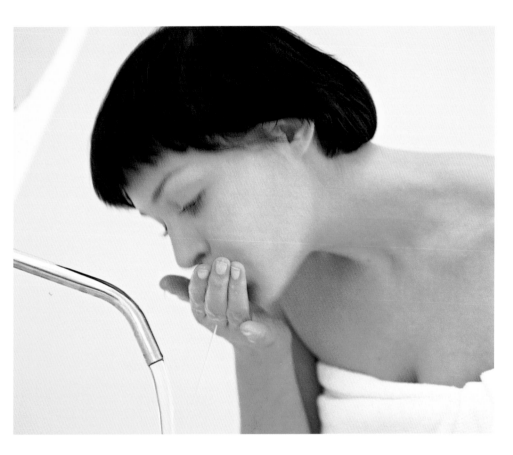

carbon molecules to bind to minerals in the body and rob it of nutrients. Even the mineral content of true mineral water is small and not always a healthy balance. If the water is high in sodium, for example, it will also have a mild dehydrating effect. On the analysis label, look for a high calcium-to-sodium ratio. If you buy bottled, go for glass, as chemicals from plastic bottles that have been left in sunlight can leak into the water.

Filtering water is another increasingly popular option. Most jug filters, which contain activated carbon and ion exchange resins, remove metals, chlorine and water hardness. But filtration also removes some of the naturally occurring minerals, such as calcium, along with the impurities.

Filters remove the chlorine put in tap water to destroy bacteria, so remember not to keep the water standing in the jug for more than a day, or be sure to refrigerate it. Also, you should change the filter regularly or the harmful residues caught inside the filter can start to leach back into the jug.

stemming the tide

It is one thing to get water into your system, another to stop it getting out. A certain amount obviously has to leave the body in order to carry away toxins and impurities. But modern living conditions encourage too much to escape. Central heating, air conditioning, sunbathing, flying, smoking, drinking and dieting are all quick routes to wrinkles.

Sunshine

If you live in the cool, dull climes of northern Europe most of the year, thank your lucky stars. You may long for more sunshine, but it comes at a cost to your skin. Warmth dramatically increases the rate of evaporation of water from the epidermis. But not only that. Sunlight sparks the production of free radicals on the skin which oxidize lipids on the epidermis and scramble up its molecular structure. Take an apple, peel it, leave it exposed to the light and it will turn brown. At the same time, its surface flesh will lose substance and tone, eventually shrouding it in wrinkles. That is oxidation – and the same thing happens to sun-drenched skin.

The sun causes 80 per cent of the changes associated with ageing. So, especially if you have dry-to-normal skin, seek the shade. If you cannot avoid or resist being in the sun, you need vitamins. Creams containing the antioxidant vitamins A, C and E have been shown to zap free radicals on contact.

Chemical sunscreen

Sunscreens, creams, blocks and lotions shield the skin from ultraviolet rays. But the more protective they become, the more they rely on synthetic chemicals. They often contain substances such as para-aminobenzoic acid, which can cause allergic eczema; stearyl alcohol, which dehydrates the skin; mineral oil, which prevents the skin breathing; methyl anthranilate, which is made from coal tar and can cause rashes; propylene glycol, which is being phased out because of adverse reactions;

alcohol, which dehydrates the skin; or courarin, which can cause contact dermatitis and photosensitivity. Among the most common side effects of sun preparations are skin burns and blisters.

Natural sunscreen

If you are exposed to only moderate sunshine and do not have fair or dry skin, a natural vegetable oil with screening properties may be enough. The most effective are jojoba, with a sun protection factor of 5–10; beeswax, which is highly viscous and sticks on the skin; and shea butter, which is 50 per cent fat, including essential fatty acids, so gives a protective seal and antioxidant protection. Avocado, rosehip, wheatgerm and sesame oils are all rich in antioxidants. You can combine these, adding vitamin E as a preservative, as in this recipe.

Sun cream

3 tbsp wheatgerm oil, 2 tbsp sesame oil or shea butter oil, 3 tbsp avocado oil, 3 tbsp jojoba oil, three capsules of vitamin E oil

Pour all the ingredients in a glass jar, put on the lid and shake well. Keep the oil in the fridge, as exposure to heat and light will destroy its antioxidant qualities. Apply it regularly to the skin in warm sun, but do not consider it complete protection. An oil like this has a sun protection factor (SPF) of 4–5, so is a sun filter rather than a block.

Smoking

After the sun, smoking is the biggest wrinkler. It thins the skin by around 40 per cent, so water escapes much more easily. Further damage is caused by chemicals that break down the fibres in collagen and elastin, accelerating the normal ageing process. Cigarette smoke contains a substance called benzopyrene which destroys the vitamin C needed for collagen manufacture and is full of free

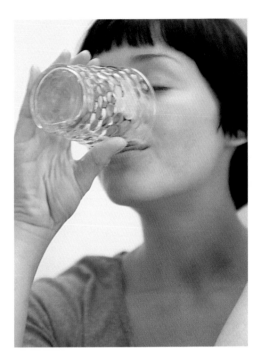

Drinking

Think how your throat and head feel the morning after you have had a drink. Alcohol dries out the skin just as much as the internal tissues that give rise to the thirst and headaches. As a diuretic, alcohol causes the body to lose water quickly. It also makes red blood cells stick together and gums up the capillaries so that they rupture, resulting in thread veins on the face. Alcohol also ages the skin by robbing the body of oxygen and vitamin C. So do your skin a favour and take up the spritzer habit.

Dieting

Losing weight is a national pastime. It is estimated that more than 85 per cent of the adult population under 50 has tried to diet. Most fail, and often harm their skin in the process. The most common mistake is to cut down on all fats. But as mentioned (see page 96) the skin relies on essential fatty acids to keep it moist and pliable. Crash dieting causes loss of muscle, which is the last thing you want if you are exercising in order to increase circulation, build muscle and maintain the hormones that benefit the skin. Yo-yo dieting (where you lose weight, regain it, lose it again and so on) has been shown to dry out and age the skin in the long term.

So if you want to lose weight but save your skin, diet at a sensible pace, include plenty of nuts, seeds and oily fish in your diet – and resolve to stick near your target weight once you have reached it.

radicals. Smoking also constricts the capillaries that feed the skin. Furthermore, the facial expressions that smoking encourages – squinting and puckering – stretch the most delicate skin on the face.

Smoking can add 15 years to the age of your skin. Smokers are five times more likely to have prominent wrinkles than non-smokers of the same age.

Central heating and air conditioning

Dehydration is the price we pay for central heating and air conditioning at home and work.

At home, keep the heating moderate and use a humidifier. A pan of simmering water or a bowl on top of a radiator are effective if less practical alternatives. Either can raise the moisture content of the air to around 80–85 per cent humidity, which is the optimal level for the skin.

Flying

The recycling of air in an enclosed cabin makes it excessively dry. There can be as little as two per cent humidity in the air and even a short flight can dry out your skin significantly. The answer is to drink water before, during and after the flight and decline alcoholic drinks.

On a long flight, take a mister and spray your face once an hour (see page 112).

make a big splash

How often have you heard someone say, 'Well, my grandmother/great aunt/mother has never used anything on her face except soap and water and she's got great skin for her age.' It is more likely to be the water than the soap that has kept her skin looking younger than her years.

Like the proverbial plant, the face benefits from external as well as internal watering. Only a small amount of fluid can be absorbed into the epidermis, whose flat, overlapping cells are at most 20 per cent water. But it can make a visible difference if they are kept at full absorption capacity. The safest, cheapest and most efficient way to do that is regularly to apply water.

Splashing your face with water not only rehydrates the skin but also stimulates the circulation. You can enhance the effect (if you dare) by using cold water or alternating cold and warm. Some people swear by a daily dousing with iced water. However, do not try that if you have very fair, sensitive skin as it may react by producing thread veins. After splashing your face, pat off only the drips and apply a water-in-oil moisturizer to control the evaporation.

But you do need to be selective about the water you use. A universal commodity it may be, but water comes in many varieties. Hard water, which contains lime and other calciferous deposits, dissolves some of the lipids on the skin's surface and disturbs the acid 'mantle' that protects it from bacterial invasion. Ideally, the skin has a pH of five to six but residues in hard water can raise its alkaline level, leaving it taut and unsupple.

If the water that enters your house is hard, tamper with it after it leaves the tap. Soluble water softeners can convert harsh, scaly water into something that your skin will appreciate. If you cannot get hold of these, use distilled or bottled water, which works out more expensive but has a similar effect.

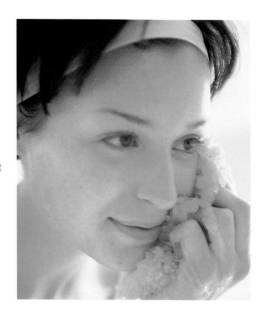

Spray away

Away from the bathroom, your face needs a portable irrigation system and appropriately, you can get one from a garden shop. A small plastic plant spray does as good a job as any of the beautifully packed 'face mister' aerosols available.

Fill the spray with distilled or bottled spring water and add up to three drops of essential oil. Floral ones such as jasmine, rose otto and lavender all work well.

Shoot the spray whenever the skin feels tight and, if flying or in very warm weather, do so regularly. Also spray your face before applying moisturizer which, as mentioned, is designed to retain existing moisture in the skin rather than add it.

Soap story

Regular splashing will rinse off some surface bacteria and grime but to do the job thoroughly you do, like your grandmother, need soap. Fortunately, soap ain't what it used to be. With a pH of 8 and a

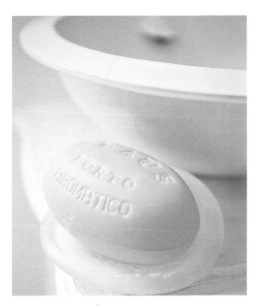

Keep it in

Ointments made from wax and oil can be used to seal in moisture and are an easy answer for dry-to-normal skin. You can make a simple version at home without the chemical preservatives that are needed in commercial moisturisers to stop the water getting infected.

Skin shield

20 g (¾ oz) beeswax, 80 ml (3 fl oz) almond or macadamia nut oil, 2 drops essential oil of rose otto

You can use almost any plant or essential oils. These are helpful because macadamia is a rich, protective oil and rose otto helps fragile capillaries. But what is most important is getting the proportions of solid and liquid fats and melting technique right.

Heat up water in a double boiler and, when the water is bubbling, put the beeswax and vegetable or nut oil in the top compartment. When the beeswax is completely melted, remove from the heat and beat the ointment until it has started to thicken and cooled to around 40–45°C (you can use a cooking thermometer to check). Then drip in the essential oil and beat thoroughly again.

Pour it into jars and store in the fridge. If your skin has an oily tendency, you may find this too sticky. If so, try 15 g beeswax to 85 ml oil and select one of the drier oils, such as thistle.

Lip lotion

20 g (¾ oz) white beeswax, 25 ml (1 fl oz) olive oil, 5 ml (1 tsp) jojoba oil, 1 capsule vitamin E, 3 drops calendula essential oil

Melt and mix the beeswax and olive oil as above. Remove from the heat, add the remaining ingredients and leave to cool in a small jar. Lavender or geranium essential oils are also good for dry or chapped lips.

fat content of only two per cent, household soap is too drying for the skin and can produce the kind of scaling and irritation that was once known as 'housewife's eczema'. The American Medical Association, in warning against the allergenic potential of many cleansers, has recommended the use of soap and water but acknowledged that it is drying to the skin.

However, you can now get a wide range of superfatted soaps (often marketed 'for sensitive skin') that contain substances such as cocoa butter or olive oil, which raise the fat level to as much as 15 per cent. Glycerin soap is also higher in fat than normal soap and benefits from the humectant property of glycerin.

Another alternative, if you want to wash with water, is to use one of the many cleansing bars or liquids available. They are made with an acid-alkaline balance much closer to the skin than normal soap and usually contain moisturizing ingredients to offset the effects of the dehydrating agents.

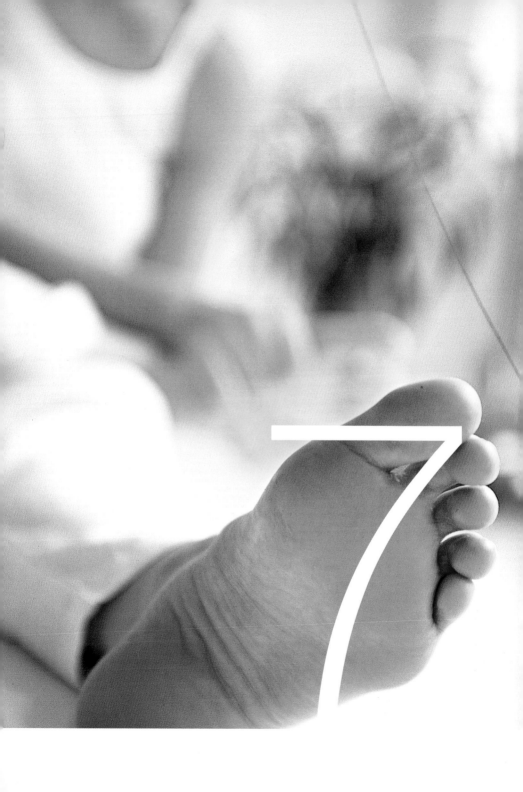

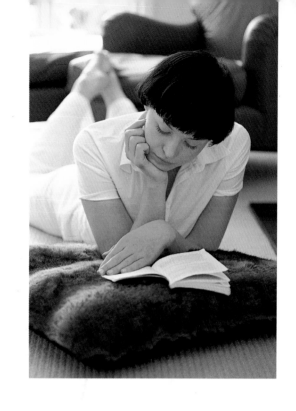

give yourself
a treat

let yourself go

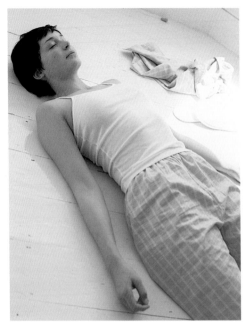

There is no hiding your problems. Your face, ever on display, is the first place to register stress. Whether it be a child struggling with her sums or an adult stuck in traffic on the way to a crucial meeting, the emotional or physical distress will be instantly visible in furrows and creases somewhere between the hairline and neck.

Everyone's face responds in a similar way. But the unfortunate difference between an adult and the child or teenager is that their skin will bounce smoothly back into place once the problem has passed. Adult skin, short on springy tissues, hangs on to the stress and embeds it deep in the dermis. The deceleration in blood flow and lymph drainage caused by the repeated stresses and strains of daily life shows not just in pallor and puffiness but in slower regeneration of cells.

Add to that the more general, long-term consequences of stress – increased blood pressure and cholesterol, lowered metabolism and immunity, blood sugar imbalance and depression – and you can see how stress adds years to your body.

Learning to relax

If the consequences of stress are complex, the solution is simple: relax. But how? It sounds so easy, yet true relaxation eludes many of us. We slump in an armchair, which strains our backs; we switch on the television, which stresses our eyes; we have a cup of coffee, which just hikes up our blood pressure.

Trying to relax, in any sense, is of course a contradiction in terms. What we need are techniques to help us release tension at will when the pressure starts to show. Many long-established and effective techniques, such as yoga and meditation, can be learnt and practised at home. Often all you need is a simple aid – a pillow, some incense, meditative music – and some peace and quiet. Others may require some input from a professional therapist.

Some therapies, such as a fingertip facelift, are applied directly to the face. Others, such as reflexology, affect the face via other parts of the body. Still others aim at an all-over relaxation which will affect your face by tranquillizing the whole nervous system. A therapy session may not come cheap, but do peace of mind and a glowing complexion have a price?

So help yourself or put yourself in the capable and calming hands of an experienced therapist. Either way, learn to relax, revive – and rejuvenate.

Strike at stress

Everyday stress is a fact of life for most people and their answer is to cope. But coping does nothing to reduce the sources of stress, so the effects are merely postponed. The answer is to learn how to manage it.

So before embarking on any specialist techniques, try to reduce the stress in your life with some simple and common-sense measures – the kind your grandmother might have issued if only you had had the time to sit down and listen to her.

First, list everything that is causing you stress and work out how to resolve each problem. Unresolved dilemmas, reinforced by lack of energy, are the major cause of stress in our lives. There is always an answer, though you may need a good friend or a professional counsellor to help you identify it.

In our 24-hour society, in which the division of labour between the genders is breaking down, lack of time is an increasingly common source of stress. How do you take the children to the swings after school when you have to rush home from work to crack on with the supper? How do you find time to buy the food for supper when you need to talk about paying the bills with your partner? How do you find time for sex when you've been watching television till midnight?

To limit, if not eliminate, the stress caused by such conflicts of interest, take these as your watchwords: prioritize, delegate, eliminate. Work out what is really important to you and what you really must (or want to) do. How many of the tasks on your list can you get someone else to do? Cross out those things that aren't essential. Leave the sheets unironed, buy a ready-cooked meal or two, decline the invitation to visit relatives. Then you may find you have time and space for positive relaxation.

Relax and revive

Achieving a fully relaxed state while remaining awake takes some conscious thought at first. But it is rather like the exercise bug: once you have experienced the daily boost it gives you, it will be a habit you find difficult to break.

Some of the most effective ways of conscious relaxation have a long pedigree, stretching back thousands of years. Yoga, meditation and visualization are three such methods that can be practised as individual disciplines or combined in your own relaxation programme. All are best learnt initially from a teacher, who can guide you on the details – such as breathing pattern, timing, rhythm and posture – that make the difference between an expedient break and a deep repose. If you don't have the time or money for that, get a self-help tape or video. Meditation (see below) is probably the easiest to try at home without any prior tuition.

Deep relaxation

Lie flat on your back with a thin cushion under your head. Stretch your arms by your sides with your palms facing up. Relax your body, limb by limb. Start with your feet, flexing your toes and letting them go; describe circles with your ankles and let them go. Tense then relax the muscles in your calves, then your thighs. Now let your spine sink into the floor and feel your abdominal muscles go. Follow the same pattern for your hands as for your feet. Allow your arms and then your shoulders to relax. Elongate then relax your neck.

Now focus on your face. Your forehead should feel completely smooth, your eyes closed, your mouth relaxed and your breath coming from deep in your diaphragm. Inhale slowly and deeply. Hold the breath. Exhale slowly. Repeat, concentrating only on your breathing, until your limbs feel floppy, your eyelids lazy and you feel totally disinclined to budge a single inch.

Meditation

Once you can achieve a deep rest using this basic pose, introduce some meditation. This does not mean immediately trying to zoom off to a higher level of consciousness on the word 'Om'. For a start, you can choose any word or sound you like; the most effective 'mantras' tend to be mono- or duo-syllabic words with an emphasis on vowel sounds. Try 'one'/ 'one-O' or 'I'/'I-ing'. The idea is to repeat the word or sound until it has pushed all other conscious thoughts from your head.

Thoughts will keep coming and going: ignore them, and always come back to your 'mantra'. Concentrate on your breathing too and eventually, conscious thoughts will be released, leading to a physical release. Your shoulders or jaw are often the first to drop. After some practice, you should feel a lot of tension dropping out of your face. You may also find that some parts of your body become numb. Enjoy these feelings, leaving the mantra echoing in your head.

If it helps, introduce some visualization. Think of a quiet stream into which your worries trickle, of a warm pink glow suffusing your body or of your tension floating away in a cloud above your head – any graphic image that helps you to imagine stress being absorbed and removed. You are using this as a relaxation technique, not a religion or policy. So do it when you can, for however long you can afford and you will appreciate the benefits more.

Exercise

Exercise seems diametrically oppposed to relaxation. But it is a short-cut to it. For exercise doesn't only boost your circulation and increase blood supply to the skin (see pages 7–9). It also burns up the residue of stress chemicals in the body while at the same time generating the production of feel-good hormones, such as endorphins, which induce relaxation.

Choose the exercise that appeals to you the most – walking, running, tennis, riding, skipping, cycling or step exercises (on and off the bottom of your staircase if you don't want to fork out for a piece of moulded plastic). Aerobic activities such as these not only build heart and limb muscle. They also increase your oxygen supply, feeding your skin and making you feel more awake, whatever you did last night. All you need to do is 30 minutes three to five times a week to make a difference.

So take regular exercise, preferably in the fresh air, but don't do it as a moral (or even cosmetic) imperative – and don't overdo it. Otherwise you will be inclined to give it up and put your feet up.

It will come as a relief to more sybaritic and less athletic readers that you don't have to don trainers or even leave your house for beneficial exercise.

Laughter and sex

Two good forms of exercise that are often overlooked are laughter and sex.

Laughing quickens your breathing, enhances the absorption of oxygen from the blood, makes your eyes sparkle by stimulating the tear glands, exercises the stomach muscles and works the facial muscles in a way that increases blood flow to the brain – all while using up 10 calories a minute. Ten seconds of a good belly laugh can raise your heart rate to the level achieved by ten minutes' rowing. In a similar way, sex boosts the circulation and triggers the release of opiates in the brain.

If they exert their effects by radically different means, what sex and laughing have in common is that both the parasympathetic nervous system into play, triggering the release of relaxant hormones and inducing tranquillity afterwards. Could you ask for more than that from an enjoyable form of exercise?

Sleep

Is any state more natural than sleep? Newborn babies can do it for anything up to 23 hours a day and many older people often seem to find it impossible to resist taking a nap in the middle of the afternoon. Yet many of us lose that innate ability to drop off at will at any time somewhere in the intervening decades.

This is as much to do with our lifestyle as any physiological changes, so you can change it. Experts have observed that, as the 24-hour society has become established, we are getting less sleep. By one estimate, our available sleeping time fell by 25 minutes over just five years in the 1990s. As ever, that deprivation shows more than anywhere in our face – in bags or dark circles around the eyes, in puffy or saggy eyelids or a drained and pallid complexion and tired-looking skin.

If you possess such undesirable features, rest assured you are not alone. The number of people seeking help for sleep problems has never been higher. The trend has led to a new branch of 'sleep medicine' and the establishment of specialized sleep clinics.

What the specialists in these clinics seek to do is monitor a sufferer's sleep pattern and diagnose the problem, from heavy snoring to an inability to switch off or waking in the middle of the night. But unless your problem is acute, you would do well first to adopt a code now known as 'sleep hygiene'. Only if your condition has not improved after a fortnight need you seek professional help.

Sleep allows the body to relax and regenerate damaged and tired cells, from your face to your feet, so adhere to the following rules to increase your quota.

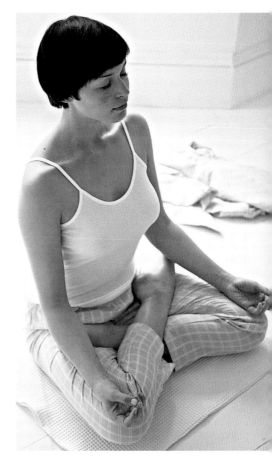

• Go to bed and get up at roughly the same time each day.
• Avoid alcohol, smoking and caffeinated drinks before you go to bed.
• Keep all work-related papers or books out of the bedroom.
• Make sure that the room is well ventilated.
• Allow yourself time to wind down before you get into bed.
• Burn a sedative essential oil in your room.
• Avoid very heavy meals in the evening.
• If you cannot sleep, sit up and read until your eyelids begin to droop. Then when you lie down, adopt the basic yoga relaxation pose to help you drop off again.

professional pampering

There is much you can do to help yourself relax. But as any infant or lover knows, there is nothing more relaxing than letting yourself go in someone else's trusted hands. The following therapies, carried out by a trained practitioner, can all lift your spirits as well as your face.

Fingertip facelift

The fingertip facelift was conceived as a natural alternative to cosmetic surgery. As such, it is non-invasive and painless. It is also supremely relaxing.

As suggested by the name, in this 'facelift' the fingers of the practitioner are the only instruments used. A form of very gentle massage is applied to increase mobility in the connective tissue, by releasing tension in the gelatin of the 'ground substance' that fills the spaces between the elastic fibres. When the gelatin is hard, practitioners say, the skin is glued to the layers of tissue surrounding the muscle and bone below. Facial mobility is decreased and creases become engraved.

By delicately manipulating the skin, the practitioner aims to unstick the gelatin and free up the muscles and connective tissue, softening and revitalizing the complexion. Some therapists incorporate into the treatment elements of acupressure and manual lymphatic drainage to enhance its effects.

A good fingertip facial can take years off you, both by relieving stress and by leaving your skin more relaxed and supple. But, as with most professional treatments, you need to have several sessions for the effect to last any length of time. Therapists also stress the importance of drinking plenty of water to keep the connective tissue soft and hydrated, and of maintaining your new-found muscle mobility with facial exercises.

Acupressure

Acupressure is based on the same principles as acupuncture. Both systems rest on the notion that energy, called 'chi' or 'qi' (pronounced 'kee'), flows through the body along invisible energy channels, known as meridians. Dotted along these, like stations along a railway line, are 'acupoints'. If there is a blockage in a point, energy cannot flow. Similarly, this causes problems further back down the line and the problem extends elsewhere in the body until the blockage is released.

The only difference from acupuncture is that, instead of stimulating the flow through these points by puncturing them with needles, acupressure works through pressure from the fingers.

By promoting good blood circulation and relieving stress, it can revitalize the skin and help to prevent bags under the eyes and wrinkles around the eyes and on the forehead. It can also relieve headache and migraine, the causes of many a furrowed brow.

In a professional treatment, the acupressurist may focus on some pressure points that are quite distant from the face, since these connect via the meridians. But because the face is at the 'end' of the body, it is the beginning and end point for many meridian pathways and rich in acupoints that you can reach yourself.

So, once you have had one or two professional acupressure sessions, you should be able to adapt the system to use on your face at home. The effect will not be as complete, but you will feel – and more importantly see – the benefits.

Self-treatment

All you need is 5–10 minutes to yourself. Put on the answerphone, remove your make-up and contact lenses and sit in front of a mirror. Work on the main acupoints, as shown opposite, progressing from the hairline down to the neck.

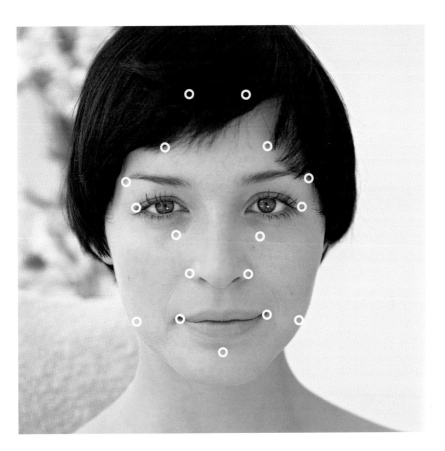

The points feel like small indentations under the skin and may feel softer or stickier than the surrounding tissue. They are quite easy to identify as each has an area into which your fingertip fits easily. Exert a light to medium pressure, ideally about 1.5 kg; you can find out how that feels by first using bathroom scales. Work in a circular motion, avoiding stretching or pulling the skin. For a lighter touch, use your third finger as it is weaker than your index finger.

There are many acupressure points on the face and neck but to simplify your self-treatment, concentrate on the nine main pairs or single points shown here. Choose those on and around the area where furrows, creases or other signs of ageing are emerging, and observe the following rules:

• Rub then shake your hands well to warm and sensitize them.

• Increase and decrease the pressure gradually at the beginning and end of each movement.

• Press for a maximum of seven seconds. If it feels uncomfortable, there is probably a blockage there and the discomfort should diminish over time. But stop if you feel pain.

Where your skin is beginning to show creases, treat the relevant points three times in each session.

Ayurvedic massage

The ancient healing tradition of Ayurveda, which means 'knowledge of life', is regarded in its Indian homeland as a blueprint for healthy living. Covering all aspects of one's physical and spiritual life, it is designed to restore harmony and vitality to the whole body.

It achieves this by incorporating many natural disciplines, such as herbalism, detoxification, nutritious diets, yoga and meditation. Ayurvedic medicine recognizes three life forces that flow through the body: vata, pitta and kapha (loosely translated as wind, fire and mucus). These three 'bioforces' are known as the tridoshas and are the basis for diagnosis and treatment.

The practitioner evaluates your constitutional type and current state of balance by reading 'the pulses' – a system of 12 positions on both arterial pulses on each wrist – to give them an understanding of the balance of the three bioforces in your overall constitution and various organs. She may also do a visual analysis, covering the tongue, fingernails, eyes, face and skin.

Treatment may include massage with appropriate oils and herbal preparations. One technique that greatly benefits the face is shirodhara, in which a head massage (see below) is followed by the drizzling of warm oil over the forehead. Continuing in a steady stream for up to an hour, it has a uniquely relaxing effect. For acute or short-term skin problems, ayurvedic herbal preparations can be very effective but always need to be prescribed by a well-trained therapist.

Manual lymph drainage

This sounds rather more like an invasive medical procedure than a beauty treatment. In fact, it is a deliciously pampering, gently pumping massage. Its aim is to drain the lymph centres of unwanted waste products that have resisted elimination through the normal channels. These wastes would otherwise remain in the body, contributing to a greyish pallor, tired eyes, puffy skin and sluggishness.

As described earlier (see pages 76–7), the lymph system relies on the contractions of muscles around the body to work. Left to itself, the lymph system may take hours, or days, to cleanse the body of wastes, and in the meantime excess fluid builds up under the skin, manifesting itself in unattractive bulges and sags. Massaging the soft tissue and muscle speeds up the release and elimination of the fluid toxins.

Manual lymph drainage can be done on the whole body – covering the many lymph nodes in the armpits and middle-to-lower trunk – or just from the shoulders upwards. The various lymph nodes of the head are each responsible for lymph drainage in parts of the face, scalp and neck.

The therapist will probably take your medical history before touching you. But once she does, you can expect to start melting into the couch. It is difficult to believe that something so effective could (totally unlike a detox diet or cold shower!) be so infinitely relaxing.

Using a variety of movements which include sweeping strokes, kneading, tapping and pressing, the therapist will apply pressure to direct the lymph fluid towards the nearest lymph node to speed up the removal of waste products. The movements vary from a deep pressure to a touch so light it barely registers.

But don't expect to get away without being given a small sermon. Manual lymph drainage is a holistic technique and therefore seen to be effective in the long term only if your habits are sympathetic to your body's needs. Your therapist will probably advise you to cut out tobacco and alcohol, for example, two of the very worst assaults made on the lymph system – and consequently on one's complexion.

Colonic irrigation

Colonics, colon hydrotherapy or colon lavage, as it is variously known, is the irrigation of the large intestine with water under gentle pressure. This clears the colon of stagnated faecal material, just as one flushes out a domestic pipe that is blocked with everyday detritus from the environment. But worry not – it is a lot gentler.

A soft, pliable tube is inserted into the anus and warm water passed up it, dislodging and diluting the waste material that travels out via the same tube. The outflow of water takes with it faeces, wind, mucus and the bacteria that grow on decomposing faeces. Devotees of colonic irrigation report feeling instantly lighter and cleaner and see a greatly improved complexion within a day or so. It is important to drink several glasses of water before and after a colonic irrigation session – but then you will be used to that anyway!

Indian head massage

This specialized form of Ayurvedic scalp massage, also known as 'champissage', is traditionally used by Indian women to keep their hair healthy and lustrous. Practitioners attribute the increasing incidence of premature greyness and baldness to tension in the head which restricts nutrition of hair follicles. Their form of head massage, which concentrates on 'marma' points on the skull similar to acupressure points, aims to relieve this tension.

But its effect on the face is equally marked, as tension in the scalp muscles is automatically transmitted to the facial muscles. By relaxing the thin layer of muscle that covers the head, a professional head massage improves blood flow to both the scalp and face.

The Ayurvedic practitioner will massage the shoulders and head for about 30 minutes, alternating firm and gentle strokes, using a warmed oil suited to the patient's constitutional type. If you carry a lot of tension in your scalp, as is very common, you may get a headache afterwards as this is released. But the visible softening of your facial contours, coupled with the deep sleep that typically follows an Indian head massage, should soon bring the smile back to your face.

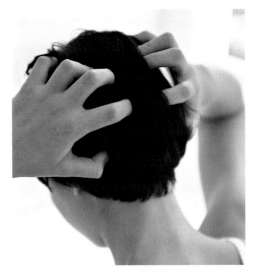

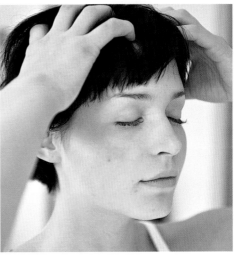

Reflexology

Reflexology, sometimes known as reflex zone therapy, is a specialized form of foot massage. The feet are about as far from the face as you could get, but reflexology is based on the principle that there are reflexes or energy channels in the feet that relate to every organ and function in the body. By applying pressure to these reflex points, practitioners believe, the energy channels in the corresponding areas are opened, restoring healthy energy flow all around the body. Muscles, including those in your face, are relaxed and the body's inherent abilities to heal itself are stimulated.

Anxiety and stress both respond very well to reflexology treatment, as do back pain, headache, migraine, blocked sinuses and circulatory problems – all of which show clearly on the sufferer's face.

After taking your medical history, the practitioner uses thumb pressure of varying strengths over the pressure points of the feet. She will concentrate on any areas that appear to be tender, as these indicate the parts of the body that need healing.

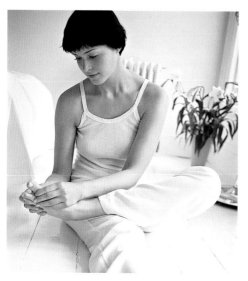

Some people find that their body goes into detox as a result of a course of treatment which, for a short while, produces aching joints, diarrhoea or a spotty complexion. Think about deferring your social engagements for a few days while telling yourself this is a good sign!

Cranial osteopathy

Cranial osteopathy, also known as cranio-sacral therapy, aims to release twisted connective tissue and compacted structure beneath the skin by restoring the body's own natural, internal rhythms. Through gentle manipulation of the skull, it aims to help the body recapture its original or optimum shape. In adults it is particularly useful for headache, migraine, dental problems, a pale or dull complexion, poor circulation and inefficient elimination. Cranial osteopathy is also used to treat poor sleep, restlessness and infections, which can equally affect the skin.

The cranio-sacral system is the core of physical life. It consists of the membranes that surround the central nervous system (the brain and spinal cord), the bones of the cranium and sacrum which attach to these membranes, the fascia which radiate out from these to all parts of the body, enveloping every nerve and nerve pathway, and the cerebrospinal fluid. Therapists believe this fluid, which is transmitted from its reservoir in the central nervous system along neurological pathways to every part of the body, carries with it a potent healing energy.

To rebalance the cranial rhythms, as they are known, the practitioner places her hands very gently on the skull and other parts of the skeletal system. This enables her to identify the areas of restriction or tension and to follow the subtle internal tugs and twists of the cranio-sacral system until points of resistance are encountered and released. Cranio-sacral therapy is generally comforting, creating a deep sense of well-being.

If you are one of the many people with a dental phobia, try hypnotherapy to banish those anxieties.

Clean your teeth night and morning, preferably with dental floss and an electric toothbrush. It takes only minutes for sugar to attack tooth enamel so also try to carry a travel toothbrush with you during the day so that you can scrub your teeth after eating anything sweet.

Additional therapies

There are many other therapies you can try that can revitalize your body from top to toe. But among those that promise to show the most in your complexion are the Bates method, Bach Flower Remedies, Reiki, Alexander Technique, Yoga, Autogenic Training, Acupuncture and Rolfing.

Laugh it off

Fastidious attention to your dental regime will enhance your smile for a while. Dedicated adherence to an exercise and massage programme that cheats time will give you a reason to keep grinning for longer. But in the end, beauty is more than skin deep. If you want to look young, don't forget to have a laugh. It's not just an antidote to the sobriety with which your appearance is now treated. Laughing will also ensure your most prominent 'dermatologic corrulations' become the irresitibly crinkly ones that everyone loves...

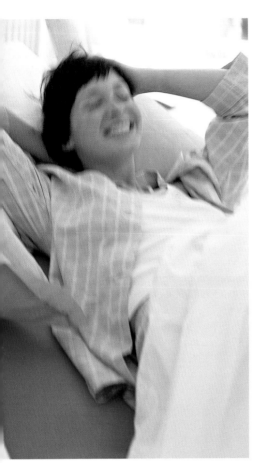

Something to smile about

There is little point in acquiring a smooth and glowing complexion if you don't have a smile to match. To avoid getting decayed or discoloured teeth, have regular dental check-ups and treatment by a dental hygienist at least every six months – more frequently if you are a smoker and/or red wine drinker as both habits stain tooth enamel. You will be much more inclined to smile once you have teeth with a sharp shine and old grey fillings have been replaced by new white ones.

give yourself a treat **125**

index

acknowledgements

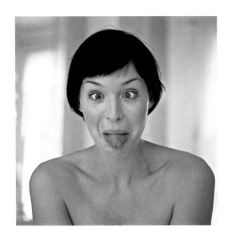

With thanks to consultants Sophie Parsons, Sebastian Parsons and Jeanette Leikauf of the Dr Hauschka skin care company for their advice on the facial exercises (pages 46–69), and Germaine Rich of Aromatherapy Associates for advice on facial massage (pages 20–45). With thanks also to the Dr Hauschka skin care company for their permission to base the facial exercises included here on those used in the Dr Hauschka Facial Gymnastics handbook.

Executive Editor: **Jane McIntosh**
Editor: **Charlotte Wilson**
Design Manager: **Tokiko Morishima**
Designer: **Ginny Zeal**
Photographer: **Bill Reavell**
Production Controller: **Nosheen Shan**
Picture Researcher: **Luzia Strohmayer**
Index: **Indexing Specialists (UK) Ltd**